Dementia: What you need to know

Dementia: What you need to know

A guide for people with dementia, and their caregivers

Dr Chris Perkins FRANZCP
Specialist in old-age psychiatry

RANDOM HOUSE
NEW ZEALAND

A RANDOM HOUSE BOOK published by Random House New Zealand
18 Poland Road, Glenfield, Auckland, New Zealand

For more information about our titles go to www.randomhouse.co.nz

A catalogue record for this book is available from the National Library of New Zealand

Random House New Zealand is part of the Random House Group
New York London Sydney Auckland Delhi Johannesburg

This edition first published 2013, reprinted 2014

ISBN 978 1 77553 482 2

Cover design: Carla Sy
Text design: Kate Greenaway

Printed in Australia by Griffin

Contents

To my mothers, Joan Arnold and Nance Perkins

Foreword

Alzheimer's is one of the words that has infiltrated our consciousness over the past decade. Along with other forms of dementia, Alzheimer's has become part of everyday conversation and concern. As life-spans lengthen, so the numbers afflicted by dementia will increase — from 35.6 million in the world in 2010 to 65.7 million by 2050. There are few of us who do not know someone with the condition, often a close relative whose loss of mental capacity is distressing to them as well as to family and friends.

But here is a book that will assist both the person with dementia and the caregiver. Life situations are always more difficult to handle in the absence of information and understanding. What is scary in the dark becomes less so when the light goes on. Chris Perkins sheds light on many aspects of dementia in this practical and compassionate book.

Understanding the nature and processes of dementia is an important start. Recognising different forms, and distinguishing it from other conditions, is an important preliminary diagnostic tool. To know the path it is likely to take is helpful in preparing for the future.

Despite common belief, the condition is not totally untreatable. Two chapters describe both medical forms of treatment and a variety of supplementary therapies that are available — massage and music, acupuncture and diet, herbal remedies and homeopathy, to name just a few. These options temper realism with hope for both the person with dementia and those who stand by.

The author deals with options for care, both residential care and care at home for the 70 per cent of people with dementia who remain in their own homes. One of the most difficult dynamics is when a caregiver has to decide when residential care is necessary, even on an intermittent basis. There is a natural sense of guilt in feeling one has failed to fully support an ageing parent. Yet the reality is that caregivers also need a break in order to care for themselves, and ultimately to be better able to care for their family member because of that.

This book explores the key topic of how one communicates with people with dementia about their condition so that a healthy and liberating transparency characterises the relationship. The discussion surrounding the tricky question of how to persuade someone to give up driving has application not just for those with Alzheimer's.

Later in the book an innovative chapter deals with the spiritual and cultural dimensions of care. In an age preoccupied with fiscal and technical criteria, it is refreshing to find attention given to those immeasurable dimensions of life that nourish the human soul. The pluralistic nature of Western society today calls for an approach that is inclusive of the spectrum of religious and non-religious spiritualities that make up our colourful communities. The author provides this with abundance.

I have known Chris Perkins for 35 years. She writes from her extensive experience as a medical professional, her own fully developed spirituality, and her deep compassion and practical wisdom. This is a book that will meet a market hungry for insights and help with a condition that leaves no family untouched. It is a pleasure to commend it as a new and accessible resource with universal appeal.

Richard Randerson

(Richard Randerson is a former Chair of the Board of the Selwyn Foundation and former Dean of Auckland Cathedral)

Acknowledgements

Some of the chapters in this book were written while I was in England in 2002. I would like to thank the staff of Sedgefield Community Hospital in County Durham for giving me the opportunity to practise in a different system with alternative approaches to dementia. I am also most grateful to Dr Alan Swann of Newcastle General Hospital in Newcastle-upon-Tyne who introduced me to all sorts of innovative ways of caring for people with dementia.

Many people have been most generous with their time, encouragement, enthusiasm and hard work in assisting in the writing of this book. Various colleagues of many disciplines read drafts and put me back on the right track when I had left it. Marie Israel, Cathy Fergusson, Margaret Wilson and Marie Todd read through the first chapters. Richard Worrall helped with behavioural and psychological symptoms, and Marion Gray with treatment. Chris Collins gave input on the caregiving chapters as did Margaret Wilson and Greg Young. John MacMillan, Bev Blake and the Counties-Manukau NASC (Needs Assessment and Service Coordination) team helped sort out the intricacies of assessment, funding and service coordination. Verna Schofield, Pat Astley, Tina Chivers, Judy Binns and Richard Worrall assisted with the residential care chapters. Bruce Connors taught me about music and art therapy. Marie Todd and Janet Turnbull contributed their expertise on geriatrics to the chapters on the final stages of the life of people with dementia. Brian Emery, Tom Rickit, Eliza Snelgar, Linda Thomson, Dr Sunita Paul, Indu Bajaj and Teuutu Pomee helped with the cultural aspects. Jean McCormick and Sue Martin reviewed the legal chapter. Stephen Jacobs spent time discussing dementia and loaded me up with information and reports. Gwendoline Smith inspired me and gave advice on the writing of books as well as sharing her own experience of coping with a loved family member with dementia. My grateful thanks to all these people. Matthew Croucher and the people at Alzheimer's Christchurch gave useful feedback on the early editions.

My 'lay' readers — sister Shirley Baddington and friends Pam Collinge and Linda, and my husband Rod — let me know when my language was too pompous, too medical or just confusing.

Barbara Smith was a wonderful support. She is an ex-caregiver to her mother with dementia, a nurse in an elderly care facility and the holder of a degree in English literature; I could not have found a more useful person to critique the drafts.

Most of all, I want to thank Jenny Taylor and her daughter Debbie, Lynley Mahon and the Wrights, who spoke frankly and movingly about their experiences of caregiving. Their stories, throughout, have added life and hope to what otherwise might be a depressing topic. I hope their bravery shines through.

I have learned most, of course, from my patients. I am truly humbled by their courage, cheerfulness and openness. I have nothing but admiration for their caregivers, who find meaning in tragic situations and continue to love and laugh regardless.

Introduction

'Alzheimer's, dementia, senility . . .' These words strike terror into the hearts of older people who have misplaced keys or forgotten the name of the person in front of them. Instantly they see their loss of memory progressing to loss of identity and total dependence on others. 'Losing our mind' means losing our selves, our dignity, our meaning and purpose and our ability to contribute. No wonder older people often say that developing dementia is their biggest worry, and the families of the person say, 'It would have been better if he had cancer.'

The fear of developing dementia is well expressed in the following letter to the editor of the *Listener*, written in support of euthanasia:

> I am an educated, strong, independent woman in my early forties. I don't want to be alive if I lose my most prized asset — my mind. I don't want to be alive if I am in a situation where I am totally reliant on others for assistance — to go to the toilet, to communicate, to turn over, to feed.[1]

When we are young, we avoid thinking about the topic altogether. When we're older, we joke uneasily about our memory lapses and avoid visiting friends with dementia. Perhaps we fear that they will somehow contaminate us, or maybe their situation is just too painful to contemplate. But dementia is here to stay. We cannot just look the other way and hope that it won't affect us. In some way, inevitably, it will . . . either as the person with it or as a carer.

The dementias are generally diseases of older people. About 5 per cent of people over 65 and 20 per cent of people over 80 are affected. In 2007, 12.3 per cent of the New Zealand population was over the age of 65 years. By 2051 this number will increase to 25 per cent. By 2035 the post-war baby boomers will be reaching age 85, so there will be a large increase in the size of the very elderly population. As our population ages, so will the number of people with dementia increase.

In New Zealand in 2011 there were approximately 48,000 people with dementia. By 2051 there will be around 50,000.[2] For each person with dementia there will be at least one or two others whose lives are seriously affected by that person's illness. Beyond that a wide circle of family, friends, professional and voluntary workers need to support the main caregiver. There is a physical and emotional toll on the carers, as well as demands on their time and loss of opportunities in other ways. Dementia is costly in the monetary sense as well, contributing to the already high health expenditure on older people. The effects of dementia spread far into the community.

Recently governments and care providers have begun to recognise that dementia is an issue that will not go away. People with dementia, including some celebrities, are beginning to speak out. Drugs that might slow or even halt the progression of the disease are being developed and we are beginning to understand how to prevent some of the disorders. There are new ways to care for and treat those suffering from these chronic brain disorders. People with dementia are being recognised as just that, people, and not as 'shells' or bodies that have outlived their brains. Communication, even with someone with very severe dementia, is possible. At another level, people are recognising that the ability to think, so highly valued by Western society, is only one aspect of being a person. Other valued actions, such as giving and receiving love, belonging to a family, being intuitive and creative, are all possible for the person with dementia.

I have written this book for New Zealanders. It is aimed primarily at caregivers and people with early dementia. It might also be useful for other people who regularly come across those with dementia. The scene is changing rapidly. Where I know that things might soon be different, I have mentioned it. Where I'm unaware of impending changes, my apologies. I view it as positive that there are so many developments going on. Hopefully all the changes are for the better!

This book is written so that it can be read straight through. However, each chapter is self-contained and can be dipped into as a reference if preferred. I may have tried to cover too much and not gone into enough depth on some subjects. I have noted (in the appendix) other resources which might be helpful for people who wish to pursue some matters further. Alzheimer's New Zealand is an excellent source of information and advice on all forms of dementia, either from its local offices or its website.

It is difficult to achieve the right balance of reality and hope. We cannot deny that dementia is a grim condition which progressively deprives people of the attributes they value. Our understanding of the different forms of dementia is nowhere near complete, and even what we do know we only imperfectly put into practice. On the other hand, attitudes have changed over the past decade and I am genuinely hopeful that people will continue to become more accepting and compassionate, offering humane and respectful care to those with dementia. If this book can do anything to reduce the stigma surrounding dementia I will be overjoyed.

We must improve the lot of people with dementia. There is a good chance that it will be our lot should we live long enough.

In his book *Dementia Reconsidered*, Tom Kitwood (perhaps the guru of dementia care) wrote in 1997:

> . . . Men and women who have dementia have emerged from the places where they were hidden away; they have walked onto the stage of history, and begun to be regarded as persons in the full sense. Dementia as a concept is losing its terrifying associations with the raving lunatic in the old-time asylum. It is being conceived of as an understandable and human condition, and those who are affected by it have begun to be recognised, welcomed, embraced and heard.[3]

References

[1] The *Listener*, 29 April 2003.

[2] *Dementia Economic Impact Report 2011*, www.alzheimers.org.nz/files/reports/Updated_Economic_Impact_Report_2012_New_Zealand.pdf

[3] Kitwood, Tom, *Dementia Reconsidered: The person comes first*, Open University Press, Buckingham, 1997.

Chapter 1
Memory and dementia

There is a wicked inclination in most people to suppose an old man decayed in his intellects. If a young or middle-age man when leaving a company, does not recollect where he laid his hat, it is nothing; but if an old man, people will shrug up their shoulders and say 'his memory is going'.

SAMUEL JOHNSON

This chapter begins with some information about memory, because poor memory is one of the main features of dementia. If we know something about memory, then we are in a better position to understand the effects its loss can have on a person's life.

Later in the chapter I will discuss the changes to memory that occur as people age, and how these differ from dementia. We will then look at the structure of the brain and how dementia is defined.

Memory

How do we remember things?

To form a memory we have to:

1. Pay attention
2. Store the memory
3. Retrieve or recall it again later.

Paying attention

We need to be alert and awake and paying attention to take things in. If we are drowsy or distracted, we do not notice what is going on around us. When we are preoccupied with worries, it is hard to take things in because our focus is on our internal thoughts. If we are totally absorbed by a novel, all sorts of things can happen without our being aware of them; later we cannot recall them. Knowing about the importance of paying attention can help to improve memory. If we can minimise distractions and focus on what we are supposed to be learning, then we are off to a good start.

Storage of memory

Immediate memory: This is a temporary storage system. We pay attention to something, for example, a phone number, use it and then forget it. If the phone is engaged and we want to try the number later, we have to look it up again. It has disappeared completely from our immediate memory. The capacity of this storage system is limited. If we try to remember both the number and something else, say, a friend's address, it is likely that the memory of the phone number will disappear.

Longer-term memory: Information has to be 'processed' to go into long-term storage. Often we process the memory by linking it to something of importance to us, for example, a topic that interests us, an emotion or a smell. This is not necessarily done consciously; however, we can use links intentionally to improve our memory — imagining a rose when we are introduced to someone called Rose. Memory improvement strategies are elaborated on in chapter 7. Memories with much emotion involved, such as a wedding day or war experiences, may be a lot more vivid and more easily recalled than everyday events.

Talking about events helps to fix them into memory. Recent memories, such as what we did yesterday, are not as well fixed in storage as older memories, like events of childhood. It seems to take some time for memories to become firmly stored.

Recall

Sometimes memories suddenly come back to us when we least expect them. The smell of sweet peas reminds me of my grandmother's garden; a hymn, the cold church and its hard seats. Sometimes, unpleasant memories come back to distress people: a car backfiring may startle a refugee and make him recall the gun battles of his home country.

'Intentional recall' is when we try to remember things from the past. This may be easier to do if there is some trigger ('cued recall'). When looking for the car keys, we might think: when did I last drive? What did I do when I came in? Where did I put my bag down? These extra details can sometimes help us to remember exactly where we left the keys. If we are trying to remember what to write in an exam, we might visualise a page of notes. Sometimes recall is effortless, but at other times it is frustratingly difficult. For some reason, when we stop trying to remember a missing fact, it will sometimes emerge spontaneously. We constantly recall things without being aware of remembering them. If we see an old school friend, we often recall their name instantly, without having to search through our memory banks.

Different kinds of memory

Personal memories: These are the things that have happened to us over our lifetimes.

Memories of places, faces and things: We recognise having been somewhere before or we know a person. We know what a thing is and what it is used for.

Procedural memories: These memories are about how to do things and are essential for our day-to-day function. They stay intact for a long time and are hard to change. (A good example of the strength of procedural memories is remembering how to ride a bicycle years after we last got on one.)

Expert memory: This is memory about things that we are skilled in, such as our job or a hobby. Some people remember complex cooking methods and recipes.

Concepts and rules: This sort of memory is about rules of grammar or arithmetic, or concepts about science or freedom of speech. If we learn them when we are young, they are hard to change.

General knowledge: Being able to recall general knowledge helps us make decisions and carry on conversations (as well as to answer questions from children).

Why is memory so important to us?

If we think about what might happen if our memory was faulty, we can understand why we need our memory in all its forms to exist in the world. Here are some examples:

Personal memory: The story of our life gives meaning to our existence and forms our character. It has an important part to play in forming our beliefs and values. Some people think our identity is lost when we forget our life history.

Memory of places, faces and things: We need memory of place to find our way around our own home, as well as the neighbourhood and the wider world. If this memory is faulty we can't go very far without getting lost. If people seem unfamiliar and we do not know their place in our lives, it can be very alarming. If we cannot both recognise a toothbrush and know what to do with it, we will need help to clean our teeth.

Procedural memory: If this is faulty we cannot function from day to day. We would need help to wash our face, tie our shoelaces, or flush the toilet.

Expert memory: Once this deteriorates we cannot continue our usual occupations. As we stop being able to do our hobbies, our lives can become boring and pointless.

Concepts and rules: It is important to comply with our society's laws and to observe social rules. If we forget what polite behaviour is, it is hard to get on in society. If we forget basic grammatical rules, people will have difficulty understanding what we are trying to say.

General knowledge: If we are unable to retain and recall general information, it is difficult to make choices. When shopping, for example, we may wish to remember the price of the baked beans in the shop down the road so we can compare it with the two different brands in another shop. This is not possible if our memory for general knowledge is lacking. A discussion may seem shallow and meaningless if a person does not recall what is going on in the world.

Immediate memory: We need this so we can make conversation or follow the plot in a TV programme. We have to be able to remember the last sentence we read for a paragraph to make sense.

New learning: Repeating what we want to know is an important part of learning. It is really difficult to learn things if we don't remember them from previous reading or learning.

Memory is vital in so many aspects of our lives that it becomes much harder to function when it is faulty.

What happens to memory in old age?

It is difficult to generalise about changes to memory in old age because everyone is different and the differences increase with age. It is hard to compare the intelligence of today's older people with younger people because of the differences in experience, education and nutrition. Research following individuals over a long period of time to see what happens to their memory is expensive, and even then changes in memory may be more to do with illness or lack of stimulation and not be directly related to age.

However, there are some age-related changes to memory that are scientifically accepted (for now).

As we age it may become harder to pay attention. We may have more difficulties shutting out external distractions (like the radio in the background). We may experience more internal distractions, such as pain or worry. Other problems, such as deafness or reduced vision, may make it difficult to receive information.

It also seems that older people are slower at processing information. They take a longer time to learn new things, and may have to ask their grandchildren to help them out on the computer or to programme the video recorder. Retrieval of information slows with age, too. This can cause problems when a person sees a familiar face but can't find the name that goes with it.

Robert Woods has some interesting statistics on age-related memory loss:

> 83% of elderly people forget names, about 60% lose keys, and about 50% cannot remember what has just been said. Only 40% forget faces or directions, and even fewer forget what they have just done, such as lock the door.[1]

Older people seem just as able as younger ones to solve problems, perhaps relying more on memory and experience than natural intelligence. Immediate memory does not seem impaired, unless there is a distraction.

The memories least likely to change are procedural memories, old personal memories, general knowledge and concepts. These are well-fixed, pre-learned items of information.

Even if we agree that overall there is some decline in intellectual ability in old age, it cannot be taken as given that any individual will show a decline. If there are memory changes, they happen so slowly that we can adjust to them and develop ways of coping so that the changes go virtually unnoticed. We carry on functioning as normal or learn to disguise the fact that we have forgotten something.

> Age is . . . practising an expansive smile at faces you've never seen that glow with recognition and chatter about familiar occasions.
>
> LATE SONG, LAURIS EDMOND [2]

The brain

The brain is divided into two main parts, the cortex and the brain stem. The part affected in dementia is usually the cortex.

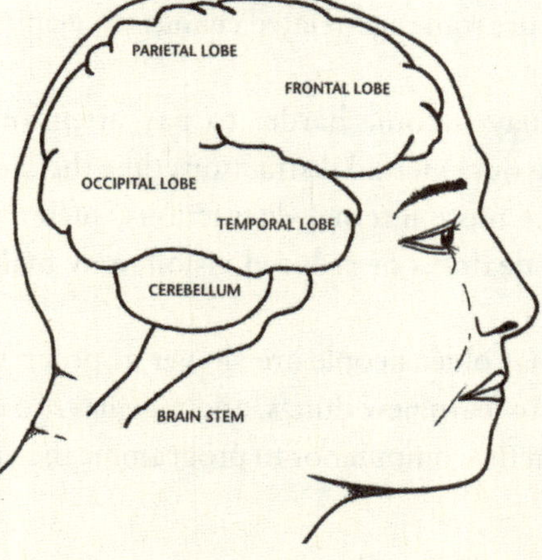

The cortex has right and left sides. Each side is divided into four main parts or *lobes*, which have different functions. The temporal lobe is thought to be the most important lobe for memory function, but the others probably also play a part in forming and storing memories.

Frontal lobes

These are at the front of the brain. They are the 'executive' lobes, meaning that they do our planning and organising. They are the last part of the brain to develop, in an evolutionary sense, and give humans the relatively bulging foreheads that make our faces look different from those of other animals. (Check your cat or dog for a forehead.)

The frontal lobes give us our personality, enable us to pay attention, solve problems, control our emotions and urges, and fit in with society. They give us the ability to weigh up competing information, desires and needs, and to make balanced judgements. Motivation and the drive to reach goals come from the frontal lobes. The frontal lobes allow us to feel and express our emotions and to be sensitive to other people.

Parietal lobes

These lobes are situated behind the frontal lobes at the top of the brain. The parietal lobes analyse information coming in from the senses (sight, hearing, touch, smell, taste and the position and internal sensations of the body). They help us put all this information together so that we understand what these messages mean. For example, they allow us to decide how far away something is that we've seen, what it is and how fast it is coming towards us. These lobes also coordinate our movements. For example, to do up a button we need to be able to see and feel the button and the buttonhole and manipulate the button so that it goes through the hole. To pick up and drink from a glass we have to be able to work out how far away the glass is (by looking at it), to know where our hand is so we can put it around the glass and where our mouth is so we can accurately move the glass to it. The parietal lobes organise these apparently simple actions so we can do them without consciously thinking. The parietal lobes also enable us to name objects, tell right from left, read, write, do maths and draw.

Occipital lobes

These lobes are at the back of the brain. Their main functions are related to vision, and include recognising objects, words, colours, movements and pictures.

Temporal lobes

The temporal lobes, situated below the frontal and parietal lobes, are important for recognising what we hear, in particular for understanding speech. The left temporal lobe is necessary for the production of speech, naming objects and remembering things we have heard. The right temporal lobe gives us musical and foreign language abilities and helps remember things we have seen. These lobes are involved in both long- and short-term memory.

Dementia can affect all areas of the cortex, though the degree to which a particular lobe is involved, and at what stage it becomes affected, depends on the particular type of dementia.

What is dementia?

Dementia is a term that covers at least 70 different illnesses that cause gradual loss of memory and other intellectual functions. Dementia usually occurs in old age, but younger people are not immune from it. Dementia is an illness. It does not occur inevitably in old age. While some changes in memory occur with ageing we must never accept that major problems with memory, thinking or function are 'just old age'. Any person with memory or thinking problems should be carefully investigated to identify the problem. They may have dementia, but the problem might be caused by another illness that can be treated.

In dementia, loss of memory (usually the retrieval and storage functions) is an important symptom, but by itself memory loss is not enough to make a diagnosis. A person with a severe dementing illness may also lose the ability to speak, write, reason, recognise things and make decisions. These are referred to as changes in cognition (thinking). There are also changes in emotion (feelings), behaviour (what people do) and perception (the way people see, hear, smell, taste or feel things). Medical people have tended to focus most on the cognitive changes, but families often find emotional, behavioural and perceptual problems the most difficult to cope with. They need help in dealing with these too.

Describing dementia

In New Zealand there are various ways of describing dementia. These different ways depend on the background of the person making the diagnosis; for example, a general practitioner, geriatrician, psychiatrist or neurologist. All agree that dementia is a neurological disorder, but each professional group puts emphasis on different aspects.

Psychiatrists commonly use the definition produced by the American Psychiatric Association in its *Diagnostic and Statistical Manual of Psychiatric Disorders* (DSM IV).[3] A simplified version is presented in the box opposite.

CRITERIA FOR DIAGNOSING DEMENTIA

Impairment of memory and one or more of the following:

- *language disturbance (aphasia)*
- *trouble carrying out motor activities (apraxia)*
- *failure to recognise or identify objects (agnosia)*
- *trouble with planning, organising things, making judgements (executive function).*

These disturbances have to interfere with work, social activities or relationships and there must be a decline in the person's functioning. Other physical and mental conditions that can look like dementia (see chapter 3) have to be excluded.

The severity of dementia can be categorised as mild, moderate or severe.

Explanation of terms used in diagnosing dementia

Memory impairment: In the early stages of dementia memory impairment is seen as forgetfulness of recent events, but as the illness progresses forgetfulness extends further and further back until the only memories left are of what happened in childhood.

Language disturbance (aphasia): Commonly people forget words and have to find a roundabout way to describe what they are talking about. A pen might become a 'writing thingy'. (This word-finding difficulty is frequent and gets progressively worse. It is not the occasional forgetting of a word, which happens to us all.)

Problems with motor activities (apraxia): People with dementia sometimes struggle to do things, such as getting dressed. Although they have no problems moving their arms or legs, they seem not to know how to use them properly. It is important to be certain a person can move their limbs before deciding they have apraxia. Stroke and arthritis can impair movement, but it does not mean the sufferer has dementia.

Failure to recognise things (agnosia): A person with dementia may have good vision yet be puzzled by a toothbrush because they no longer know what it is for. Similarly, someone with agnosia may put a video cassette in the microwave because they cannot identify what items are supposed to go where.

Failure of executive function: A person with dementia may lose their ability to organise, sequence, think abstractly, make judgements. Preparing a meal takes a great deal of coordination and planning. A previously efficient cook who develops dementia may have the potatoes cooked half an hour before the meat is ready and have not yet turned on the vegetables (showing poor planning and sequencing). A person with poor executive function may not understand the reasons for paying taxes (doesn't understand abstract concepts) or may sell his house for a ridiculously low price (showing poor judgement).

If the changes are so slight as to not interfere with the person's life in any way, the person is not considered to be suffering from an illness. Also, a person may have had lifelong problems with planning and organising things. Only if this has become worse should it be considered to be a symptom of dementia.

Severity of dementia

In mild cases of dementia, though work or social activities are significantly impaired, people can still live independently. For example, they can keep themselves clean, feed and dress themselves, cook and manage money.

If the dementia is moderate, independent living is risky and some supervision is required. People might forget to take their pills, occasionally burn pots or give large sums of money to the local children.

People with severe dementia need continual supervision. They need help to shower and get to the toilet. Their speech may deteriorate to the point that they can't be understood.

Problems with the DSM IV diagnosis

This definition (along with others) is not entirely satisfactory for the following reasons:

1. Memory loss is the main symptom of most dementias and the DSM IV diagnosis cannot be made without it. However, sometimes the memory loss is the least of a person's worries. It is not always the first problem to surface and other major problems may arise before memory goes. In the frontotemporal dementias, memory loss may occur very late.

2. The DSM IV notes that there may be problems with behaviour, mood and delusions (false beliefs) but does not include these in the definition itself. Changes in personality are not mentioned either. Some people think the definition focuses too much on the cognitive (thinking) changes and does not adequately acknowledge the other problems associated with dementia.

3. Unless the symptoms cause problems in functioning in some way, a diagnosis of dementia is not made. In the early stages of the illness, these

problems may be very subtle or compensated for by the person, but there is still a possibility that they have dementia and might benefit from treatment.

Nevertheless, the DSM IV definition is an adequate description of the symptoms that most people get. It describes something different from the milder memory problems that occur normally as we age, in that there are more areas of thinking affected.

The fifth version of the DSM (DSM V) is now being developed. The term 'dementia' will be replaced with 'neurocognitive disorder' — mild or major. The proposed criteria are: problems with attention, executive ability, learning, memory, language, visiospatial skills and social understanding. We will have to wait and see whether these are an improvement on DSM IV. Will it be better or worse to have a diagnosis of 'neurocognitive disorder' than 'dementia'?

In the next chapter we look at the different types of dementia.

References

1 Woods, Robert T. (ed.), *Psychological Problems of Ageing, Assessment, Treatment and Care,* Wiley, New York, 1999.

2 Edmond, Lauris, 'This year 1000 Americans will live to be over 100', in *Late Song*, Auckland University Press, Auckland, 2000, p. 32.

3 *Diagnostic and Statistical Manual of Psychiatric Disorders*, 4th edition, The American Psychiatric Association, Washington, 1994.

Chapter 2

Types of dementia

In completing one discovery we never fail to get an imperfect knowledge of others of which we could have no idea before, so that we cannot solve one doubt without creating several new ones.

JOSEPH PRIESTLEY

There are many forms of dementia. In this chapter we focus on the more common types. These are:

- Alzheimer's disease: accounts for (roughly) 60 per cent of all dementias
- Vascular dementia: 10–20 per cent of dementias
- Mixed Alzheimer's disease and vascular dementia: about 10 per cent of dementias
- Lewy body dementia: 10–15 per cent of dementias
- Frontotemporal dementia: about 10 per cent of dementias.

It is not always possible to diagnose exactly which form of dementia a person is suffering from. To complicate matters, experts disagree about the classification of the dementias. Does frontotemporal dementia really exist as a separate entity or is it just an unusual manifestation of Alzheimer's disease or vascular dementia? Is Alzheimer's disease actually a form of vascular dementia? Is Alzheimer's one disease or many disorders that look roughly similar? How does Lewy body dementia relate to the dementia sometimes seen in Parkinson's disease? Is it the same thing? These are just some of the questions that challenge dementia researchers today.

Although it is frustrating not to have a cut-and-dried understanding of the dementias, the debate is a sign of increased interest and research in the area. People can no longer be told 'it's just old age' or given the label 'senile' when there are descriptions of definite patterns of disease and ideas of how to treat each one.

Alzheimer's disease

What it looks like

One of the earliest signs of Alzheimer's disease is loss of short-term memory. With this comes difficulty recalling what one has been told, asking the same questions over and over again, forgetting appointments and leaving pots on the stove to burn dry. These things also happen to people who don't have dementia but who are preoccupied with other things, or just not paying attention to what they're doing. However, in Alzheimer's disease, the person's memory gets progressively worse and other skills are gradually lost. Problems with speech, depth perception (judging how far away things are) and direction finding may occur early in the illness. The person usually retains good social skills and personality does not change a great deal until late in the illness.

Because the changes are so gradual it is often difficult to decide when they started. People sometimes date the onset of Alzheimer's to a time of stress such as a partner dying or a physical illness. They believe that the stress caused the memory decline. However, often, on careful reflection, it can be seen that the person was unable to cope with the changes foisted on them by the crisis because they had problems thinking and could not adapt to a new situation. Frequently a husband or wife has compensated for the failing memory of their spouse, so the memory problem was not apparent until that person died or went into hospital, leaving the impaired partner alone. The person with dementia could cope with an established routine and familiar surroundings, but becomes confused in a changed situation, a different environment or if there are new tasks to learn. The following example shows how illness may be hidden from the outside world.

Mr and Mrs A. lived a self-contained existence. He had heart failure and his shortness of breath made it difficult for him to move round, but he could tell Mrs A., who had memory problems, what to do to help him. Mr A. never wanted any outside help, saying they could manage on their own. They did manage reasonably well for years.

One morning the neighbours found Mrs A. wandering in the garden in a distressed state. She couldn't tell them what was the matter, but eventually they went into the house and found that Mr A. had died, apparently in his sleep.

Mrs A. could not tell the neighbours the phone numbers of her children and she was unable to make any decisions about the funeral. The neighbours initially put this down to shock but soon realised that Mrs A. was quite disabled and arranged to have people stay with her to keep her safe.

The course of Alzheimer's disease

The characteristic course of Alzheimer's disease is slow and relentless. There is a gradual decline in cognitive ability accompanied by loss of skills. Later there may be behavioural difficulties and psychological problems such as delusions (false beliefs) and hallucinations (seeing or hearing things that aren't there). In the final stages the person is unable to walk or talk and is totally dependent on others. As a rule, the older the person is when it starts, the slower the disease progresses. As a rough guide, for a person over 70, it is two to seven years before the diagnosis is made (mild illness); this is followed by four to five years during which the person can manage at home (mild to moderate illness) and two to three years in care (severe illness). This gives a time course of eight to seventeen years overall. In younger people it often has a much faster course. More detailed descriptions of the course of Alzheimer's disease and the other dementias are given in chapters 4, 5 and 6.

Who gets Alzheimer's disease?

It is mostly older people who suffer from Alzheimer's disease; the average age of onset is 78. However, this does not mean that people under 65 years are immune from it. People with a lower educational level seem more likely to get Alzheimer's. Women have a slightly higher incidence of the disorder than men. This holds true even when account is taken of their longer life expectancy, different educational history, smoking, head injury and the like. There are some families where many members develop an early-onset form of the disease. Familial Alzheimer's is rare, affecting only about 2–3 per cent of people with the disease. (Because Alzheimer's disease is very common, most people will have a relative with the disorder. If this is true for you, it does not mean your chances are higher than anyone else's for getting the disease.) People with Down's syndrome, a common form of intellectual disability, are particularly susceptible to Alzheimer's, which frequently begins when they are in their 40s or 50s. People with a relative who has Down's syndrome also have an increased incidence of Alzheimer's. Having a serious head injury may make people more prone to this disease. Recent research has shown that treating people's high blood pressure reduces the incidence of Alzheimer's disease. This suggests that people with hypertension may be at risk of getting this form of dementia as well as vascular dementia. Many other possible predisposing causes — from smoking, to oestrogen deficiency, to nose picking (it might introduce infection) — have been investigated but no link has been found to date. High blood levels of aluminium can cause a form of dementia, but this is not Alzheimer's disease. Certain viruses can cause some forms of dementia, but there is no evidence to link them with Alzheimer's disease.

Genetics

Because Alzheimer's disease can occur in families and is frequent in people with Down's syndrome (a condition caused by a faulty chromosome), people began to look for a gene that might be associated with Alzheimer's disease. Genes could cause Alzheimer's-type dementia, increase the risk of developing the illness or make it come on at an earlier age.

In Down's syndrome there are problems with chromosome 21 or, more rarely, 14 or 19. Alzheimer's researchers, following the lead from Down's syndrome, have found at least six different chromosome abnormalities that may cause the typical changes of Alzheimer's disease in the rare inherited cases. There are abnormalities on chromosomes 1, 14 and 21 that cause alterations in the way we make some proteins. This causes excessive amounts of a protein called amyloid to be deposited in the brain. Amyloid deposits may damage the brain and cause the visible changes of Alzheimer's disease.

Some genes that don't cause Alzheimer's but may make people more prone to developing the illness have also been detected. The relevant genes are called 'ApoE'.

- ApoE 2 gene appears to protect people from getting Alzheimer's.
- ApoE 4 is thought to bring the onset of the disorder ahead by 4–5 years.
- ApoE 3, the most common ApoE type in the population, appears not to influence the development of Alzheimer's disease.

Knowing that someone is slightly more likely than other people to get Alzheimer's disease is not particularly useful information, given the absence of any form of prevention (apart from healthy living). Even in the early-onset, hereditary form of the disease, individuals already know that they are at increased risk. In Sweden, when members of affected families were offered genetic testing, very few accepted the offer, preferring not to know either way.

In cases where an individual is already exhibiting symptoms, the test could be useful. The current accuracy of diagnosis made from clinical history, examination and tests is about 80–85 per cent. Knowing that the person has ApoE 4 increases the accuracy to about 90 per cent. ApoE testing in New Zealand is performed at Christchurch Hospital, but as you can see, the test by itself is not very good at predicting Alzheimer's disease. Genetic studies are still in the very early stages. They will add to our understanding of Alzheimer's disease and we hope, in future, help to prevent or treat the condition.

For a 2008 update, see www.alzheimers.org.uk/factsheet/405

What happens in the brain?

Under the microscope

In 1907, when Alois Alzheimer examined the brain of his patient, Augusta, under the microscope, he saw what he described as plaques and tangles. These are the characteristic signs of Alzheimer's disease. We now know that plaques are made of the protein amyloid; the tangles are parts of dying nerve tissue. These develop in normal brains with age, but are much more numerous in Alzheimer's disease. The damaged nerve cells also contain abnormal proteins, called tau and ubiquitin. More recently pathologists have found signs of inflammation in the brain, especially around the blood vessels. As the nerve cells die, the brain shrinks. The temporal lobes, which deal with memory, are especially affected.

Chemical changes

Healthy brain cells produce neurotransmitters. These are chemical 'messengers', which are released from the ends of nerve cells in the brain to carry information to the next nerve cell. Memory and other brain functions depend on these messengers. There are hundreds of different neurotransmitters, but the one that we know most about in Alzheimer's disease is acetylcholine. In Alzheimer's disease there are low levels of acetylcholine in the hippocampus and the amygdala, areas important for memory. Understanding about the lowered brain levels of acetylcholine has led to the development of the first specific treatments for Alzheimer's disease. More recently there has been interest in a similar neurotransmitter, butyrylcholine, which is also depleted in Alzheimer's patients.

If we knew why these physical and chemical changes occurred, we might be on the way to preventing this illness. We do know it is not just ageing, because not everyone develops Alzheimer's disease, even those who live to a very great age.

What tests are available for Alzheimer's disease?

Unfortunately, despite the increased knowledge about what is going on in the brain, there is still no definitive test for the disease. Even brain biopsies (taking a small piece of tissue out of the brain and examining it under the microscope) do not give a definitive diagnosis and, unsurprisingly, are not done very often. However, by talking to a patient and their family, doing a physical examination and tests to make sure nothing else is going on, an experienced doctor can make a diagnosis with reasonable accuracy (80–85 per cent). Perhaps people are a little less trusting of this way of making a diagnosis than they used to be. They would like to have a blood test or an X-ray that told them 'Yes, you definitely have Alzheimer's disease' or, preferably, 'No, you don't'.

Research to find a reliable test is continuing. Possibilities include special scans of the brain and more sophisticated genetic testing. Psychological tests can help in doubtful cases, but these take several hours and are tiring for the patient. So far, there is no one test or simple procedure that is totally reliable.

Can Alzheimer's disease be prevented?

As yet we don't have any known way to stop people getting this illness. Many preventative strategies have been suggested, but there is no proven method. A good education seems to be preventative.

The current suggestions on how to reduce dementia risk (from Alzheimer's Australia's 'Mind Your Mind' website) are:

1. Mind your brain — by keeping mentally active with new learning puzzles, hobbies and cultural activities.
2. Mind your diet — reduce saturated fats and eat unsaturated fats, Omega-3 fatty acids (in soy, canola and flaxseed oils, and fish), antioxidants (dark vegetables, green tea, etc.), folate and vitamins E and B12.
3. Mind your body — exercise regularly, including weight training, balance and aerobic fitness.
4. Mind your health checks — check blood pressure, cholesterol and blood sugar levels and avoid obesity.
5. Mind your social life — keep in contact with family, friends, neighbours, clubs and social groups. Get involved in community work.
6. Mind your habits — don't smoke, don't drink too much and get plenty of sleep.
7. Mind your head — avoid head injury by taking sensible precautions.

There are no specific drugs (other than those to treat hypertension, diabetes and high cholesterol) to reduce risk. Some research suggests that anti-inflammatory drugs, such as aspirin, Brufen and Voltaren, taken for long periods earlier in life might reduce the incidence. Oestrogen taken as hormone replacement therapy does not help and can have serious side effects.

Research

The new gene therapies, when they become available, may be used to prevent the onset of Alzheimer's, especially in people with a strong family history of the disease.

Vaccines: Anti-amyloid immunisation has been tested in animals and seems to successfully prevent the development of amyloid plaques. There are problems, though, because the vaccine causes inflammation of the brain. So there is more work to be done there!

As is obvious from the above list, it is the same old story! Look after your health, eat plenty of fruit and vegetables, exercise your brain and body, and don't do things that might cause head injury. Get your blood pressure, weight, blood sugar and lipids down to near normal. There are some other possibilities in the wings, but they are not certain enough to spend a lot of money on just yet.

Vascular dementia

The word 'vascular' applies to the blood supply. In vascular dementia, there is inadequate blood supply to the brain. As cells are starved of oxygen and nutrients (especially glucose, which is the brain's energy source), they die.

Disruption of the blood supply to a brain cell can be chronic or acute. In the chronic state, a blood vessel gradually narrows and doesn't supply quite enough blood for the cell's needs. This slow starvation causes ischaemic cell damage. Sudden, acute damage occurs when there is an abrupt blockage of a blood vessel by a blood clot. If the blocked vessel is quite large, the brain damage is evident as a stroke (also known as a cerebrovascular accident, CVA), which typically presents as one-sided weakness, changes in speech or other problems. A temp-orary CVA, known as a transient ischaemic attack (TIA) may briefly cause slurred speech, loss of balance or loss of consciousness. This occurs when the blood supply is temporarily disrupted; but flow is restored when the clot breaks up or another blood vessel opens up to supply the affected area. Whether the loss of blood supply is sudden or gradual, eventually enough brain damage occurs from cell death for it to be noticeable as vascular dementia. A person can have both vascular dementia and Alzheimer's disease — this is called mixed dementia.

What it looks like

Vascular dementia is much more variable than Alzheimer's disease. Different parts of the brain are affected depending on which areas have lost their blood supply, so there is a patchy pattern of change in thinking. For example, if the frontal lobe is affected, the person might not make very good decisions. If the parietal lobe is damaged, the person might have trouble with numbers or recognising objects.

In vascular dementia, the criteria for diagnosing dementia must be met (poor memory, changes in thinking, loss of function etc.), but there will also be other signs or symptoms suggesting damage to various areas of the brain. These features may include early changes in walking (gait disturbance), early development of urinary problems such as incontinence, symptoms suggestive of Parkinson's disease and other abnormal signs found on testing.

The course of vascular dementia

The course of vascular dementia may be smoothly progressive if there is a gradual cut-off of blood supply. Alternatively, there may be a sudden decline and then a levelling out for a period, then another sudden deterioration. These abrupt downward steps correspond to 'mini-strokes' occurring when a tiny blood vessel is blocked and a little brain tissue dies. There is no particular time course for vascular dementia. A person may survive up to 20 years after dementia is recognised or might die much sooner from a stroke or problems related to poor blood supply to other organs such as the heart.

Who gets vascular dementia?

Anyone who has a condition that causes damage to blood vessels is at increased risk of getting vascular dementia. Damage to blood vessels can result from:

- High blood pressure (hypertension)
- Diabetes
- Elevated blood lipids, including cholesterol (hyperlipidaemia)
- Smoking
- Family tendency to vascular disease.

There are other conditions that make an individual more prone to vascular dementia. Two such conditions are irregular heart rhythms (usually atrial fibrillation) where there is a risk that clots will travel from the heart to the brain, and certain blood disorders where the blood is much more likely to clot than normal.

Generally, men are more likely than women to suffer from vascular dementia. Some studies have shown that vascular dementia accounts for 60 per cent of dementia in people of Asian ethnic background, but there are now doubts as to the accuracy of these figures. Maori and Pacific Islanders may have a relatively higher rate of vascular dementia because they are more prone to the underlying conditions that damage blood vessels. Vascular dementia tends to start at a younger age than Alzheimer's disease.

Genetics

The genetics of vascular disease are the same as those of the underlying conditions. High blood pressure, diabetes and hyperlipidaemia often run in families, but not always.

What happens in the brain?

The carotid arteries that run up the neck supply blood to the brain. Once inside the skull, the arteries branch and continue to divide into smaller and smaller vessels (like tree branches) to supply the brain tissue.

The usual cause of damage to arteries is arteriosclerosis, which is the stiffening of the blood vessel wall and roughening and narrowing of the inside of the artery. Imagine the artery as an elastic pipe. The stiffening of the wall makes it harder for the vessel to respond by expanding or contracting to changes in blood pressure. Blood pressure is changing all the time in response to activity, posture, emotion and other factors. Blood vessels narrow or open up to keep the pressure at the right level. If blood vessels can't respond, the brain may be starved of blood or get too much blood. A drop in blood pressure may mean there is not enough blood supplied to the brain cells. Sudden rises in blood pressure can break the delicate blood vessel walls and cause bleeding in the brain, which damages cells.

Inside, the artery is furring up like an old pipe, so there is less space for the blood to flow through. If the inside lining of the artery is rough, clots can form on the walls. These clots can later break off and lodge further along the artery where it narrows, so blocking blood flow.

The brain cells die, the tissue scars or turns to liquid. Over time this becomes widespread and the brain becomes riddled with holes and scars and it shrinks. It is likely that (as in Alzheimer's disease) the production of the neurotransmitter acetylcholine diminishes.

What tests are available for vascular dementia?

The patient's history and a clinical examination remain reasonably good tests for vascular dementia. However, CT (computerised tomography) and MRI (magnetic resonance imaging) scans can show up specific vascular damage, such as the fluid-filled holes called lacunae (Latin for lakes) and white matter hyperintensities (areas of brightness), which indicate poor blood supply. These hyperintensities are often at the end of the distribution network of the blood vessels, so they form a characteristically recognisable pattern.

Of course, it is never that easy! An MRI scan of the brain of a perfectly normal older person will show changes like this, but the degree of change is usually less than is seen in cases of dementia. Like most other tests in medicine, a scan will only confirm what is already suspected. Finding vascular changes doesn't rule out co-existing Alzheimer's disease; mixed dementia is not uncommon.

Can vascular dementia be prevented?

Factors that damage blood vessels can cause vascular dementia. Prevention means not smoking and getting treatment for high blood pressure, diabetes and high blood lipids. This is not always as straightforward as it sounds. If blood pressure drops too far ('hypotension') or blood sugar is too low ('hypoglycaemia'), then brain cells will be damaged. To be on the safe side, doctors often aim to keep the blood sugar of diabetic older people just a little higher than normal.

The other treatment commonly used to prevent vascular dementia is the humble aspirin. Taken in small doses of 75–150 mg or 1/4 to 1/2 of a standard 300 mg tablet, this stops platelets, the clotting cells in blood, from sticking together. Though there is still some debate about its usefulness, aspirin is cheap and usually safe enough for most people. Its main side effect is that it can irritate the stomach lining, causing bleeding. This can be overcome by taking specially coated tablets. However, some people are allergic to aspirin-type drugs and cannot take them at all.

Mixed dementia

Mixed dementia is a combination of both Alzheimer's disease and vascular dementia, but it may look like either form of dementia.

Lewy body dementia

Lewy body dementia has been recognised only since the mid-1990s. It may account for about 10 per cent of cases of dementia. It seems to be closely related to Parkinson's disease, because people with Lewy body dementia have physical symptoms suggestive of Parkinson's disease, and people with Parkinson's disease often develop a type of dementia.

The boundaries between Lewy body dementia and Parkinson's disease with dementia are, as yet, indistinct. Generally we diagnose a 'Parkinson's dementia' if the Parkinson's symptoms have been present for a year before the dementia occurs.

What it looks like

In Lewy body dementia memory loss may not appear as early as in Alzheimer's disease. The initial deterioration is in the person's ability to pay attention and evidence of trouble with spatial tasks, such as judging depth, recognising objects and making or copying three-dimensional figures. The other symptoms of dementia follow.

Characteristically, a person's abilities fluctuate; a person will appear more alert and aware at one time and more confused at another. The person may actually lose consciousness and repeated falls are not uncommon. These could result from changes in consciousness or from a loss of blood pressure control as a result of which the person's blood pressure drops when they stand up (orthostatic hypotension). Another hallmark of Lewy body dementia is the presence of hallucinations. With visual hallucinations a person sees, sometimes quite vividly, things that are not there, often people or animals. Auditory hallucinations (hearing noises or voices not audible to others) are much less common. Hallucinations can be very disturbing and the person may act in response to them. Alternatively, the person may be indifferent to them or even amused by them. Parkinsonian symptoms of Lewy body dementia include stiffness (rigidity) and changes in posture (which becomes stooped) and walking (the person shuffles or gets 'stuck'). The person's face may become wooden and expressionless, as occurs in Parkinson's disease. Along with this the person will be very sensitive to antipsychotic medication (which is used to treat such symptoms as hallucinations), responding with markedly increased rigidity.

The course of Lewy body dementia

The course of the disorder is similar to Alzheimer's disease. There are usually several years before diagnosis, followed by three to four years at home and then one to two years in care. While the course is progressive in that cognitive function and skills gradually diminish, the fluctuations of the illness may mask this.

Who gets Lewy body dementia?

This is a disorder of older people, although the youngest reported case began at the age of fifty. Slightly more men than women get Lewy body dementia. People with Parkinson's disease who develop dementia are likely to get the Lewy body type. Other than this, we don't know who else might be predisposed to getting it.

Genetics

We don't know much about the genetics of the disease, either. There are some forms of Parkinson's disease that run in families. Whether this is true also for Lewy body dementia is, so far, unclear. There is an increased proportion of people with the ApoE 4 type of gene, as in Alzheimer's disease, but we do not know whether this means the two disorders are related.

What happens in the brain?

Lewy was a student of Alzheimer. In 1912 he identified some abnormal microscopic bodies in the brain cells of people with Parkinson's disease. These so-called Lewy bodies occurred in the sub-cortical part of the brain, which is involved in movement, balance, posture and consciousness. It is the non-thinking part of the brain that nevertheless is essential for keeping us breathing, walking and coordinated. Lewy bodies in the sub-cortical region were thought to be part of the problem in Parkinson's disease.

Much later, these Lewy bodies were rediscovered, this time in the cortical area of the brain, where thinking and memory occurs. They also occur in normal older brains, but are much more prominent in people with Lewy body dementia. As in Alzheimer's disease there are plaques, but not many tangles. Thirty per cent of people with Lewy body dementia also exhibit signs of vascular change.

As in the other dementias, the cells die and the brain shrinks, though the pattern of shrinkage is different from that seen in Alzheimer's disease. Levels of acetylcholine are very depleted in this disorder, as are those of the neurotransmitter dopamine. The lack of this latter chemical causes symptoms of Parkinson's disease.

What tests are available for Lewy body dementia?

There are no particular tests for the diagnosis of Lewy body dementia. Again, like Alzheimer's disease the diagnosis is made from the history (that is, the development of the problems and their pattern) and a clinical examination. If a CT scan of a person with Lewy body dementia is compared with one of Alzheimer's disease, generalised shrinkage is seen in both, but the medial temporal lobes, which are especially affected in Alzheimer's disease, are not so damaged in Lewy body dementia.

Not many New Zealand radiologists (the people who read the scans) are experienced in measuring the relative size of the medial temporal lobe, but interest in this area is growing.

Can Lewy body dementia be prevented?

We do not yet understand enough about the Lewy body dementia to know how to prevent it.

THE COURSES OF DIFFERENT TYPES OF DEMENTIA

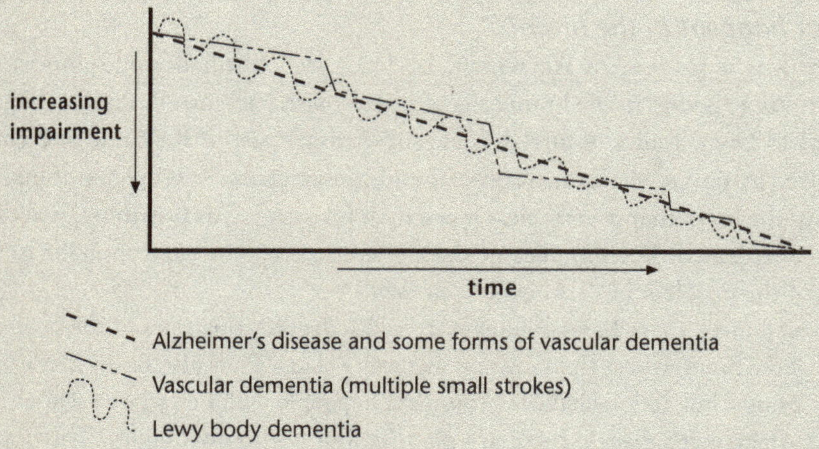

Frontotemporal dementia

Frontotemporal dementia is a group of disorders, rather than one single disease. What they have in common is damage to the frontal lobes of the brain and often the temporal lobes as well. They account for maybe 10 per cent of dementia cases in the elderly and 20 per cent in people younger than 65. The function of the frontal lobes has been discussed in chapter 1. This is where the delicate and intricate systems responsible for our more sophisticated behaviour as human beings are located.

About 100 years ago Arnold Pick described an illness that caused degeneration of the frontal and temporal areas of the brain and showed characteristic changes on autopsy. Pick's disease was thus the first frontotemporal dementia to be recognised. Subsequently, people have discovered many other forms of frontotemporal dementia.

Types of frontotemporal dementia

- Pick's disease
- Familial frontotemporal dementia (rare diseases that run in families)
- Semantic dementia (speech is affected first)

- Primary progressive aphasia (speech is the main problem)
- Traumatic brain damage (from head injury)
- Alcohol dementia or dementia resulting from other toxic substances
- Dementia associated with movement disorders; for example, Huntington's and motor neurone disease (sub-cortical changes occur first, though)
- Dementia associated with other brain disease; for example, Alzheimer's disease and vascular dementia.

What frontotemporal dementia looks like

There are distinctive features that make frontotemporal dementia recognisable. These are changes in behaviour, personality, emotion and speech, which occur despite other cognitive functions (such as memory, spatial skills and ability to recognise things) remaining initially unchanged.

Behaviour and personality changes: People suffering from frontal lobe problems may become tactless and not conduct themselves in the manner expected in a particular social situation. They may neglect personal hygiene or dress oddly. Sometimes they lose their inhibitions so that they take uncharacteristic risks or behave in a sexually inappropriate way. A previously introverted person might become unusually outgoing. All this can be acutely embarrassing to friends and family, but the person with frontotemporal dementia is blithely unaware of these effects. This loss of understanding that anything is wrong (loss of insight) occurs early on in the disease.

The case below shows how such behaviour may manifest. Initially, it was hard to decide what was wrong with this lady.

> *Mrs W.'s daughters took her to the GP because they were alarmed by her unusual behaviour. The doctor realised there was something really wrong when Mrs W. walked straight into his office while he was examining another patient. He thought she needed to see an old age psychiatrist and referred her to me.*
>
> *When Mrs W. came to see me, she got up and left the room as soon as she had finished talking. She seemed unaware that there are certain social conventions associated with a visit to the doctor (like waiting to discuss the diagnosis and treatment) and leave-taking (excusing yourself, saying goodbye).*

The behaviour of a person with frontotemporal dementia might become rigid, so the person finds it difficult to accept new ideas or to change from a routine. Or behaviours may become repetitive, the same thing being done pointlessly over and over again (such as clapping or repeatedly going to the toilet). On the other hand, people with frontotemporal dementia may be easily distracted from a task and never complete anything.

Sometimes people with this disorder feel the urge to have things in their mouths and will always be eating, smoking or drinking, or even putting inedible things in their mouths. They may develop a liking for sweet foods. They will explore objects in their environment with their hands as well, and try using them in a variety of ways for which they weren't intended.

Emotional symptoms: People with frontotemporal dementia can become depressed, anxious or excessively sentimental. Often their emotions are not the right ones for the situation, such as laughing on sad occasions. Suicidal thoughts and delusions (false beliefs) can occur. People with frontotemporal dementia may be overly concerned about their health. Or they may lack emotional expression altogether, seeming not to have feelings. They are often unaware of or unsympathetic to the feelings of others. They can become passive, not initiating or wanting to do anything, though they will go along with what others organise for them.

Speech disorder: They may be unable to recall the right word for the situation, or use many words without conveying much information. Alternatively, the amount of speech might be reduced or they might just say the same words or get stuck on a single theme. Sometimes they pointlessly repeat what someone else has just said. In the later stages, speech is totally lost.

In progressive aphasia, an effort is required to produce speech and the person has trouble finding words. There are errors in grammar and the way words are pronounced, and reading and writing might be difficult. The person, however, can still understand what is said.

In semantic dementia, the main problems are in naming things and understanding speech.

The course of the disorders

The course of a frontotemporal dementia depends very much on its cause. The time from onset to death can range from two to more than ten years. If it is a primary frontotemporal dementia (that is, not one caused by Alzheimer's or vascular dementia), the person is unlikely to have severe memory problems early on. These develop later and the disorder begins to look more like Alzheimer's disease. If the frontotemporal dementia is caused by an injury to the brain, it may remain static for decades. If the damage has been caused by excessive alcohol, its progress can be slowed or at least partially reversed by abstinence.

Who gets it?

Pick's disease and the familial frontotemporal dementias classically begin between the ages of 45 and 65 years. However, these disorders can develop in old age. Equal numbers of men and women are affected. People with motor neurone disease or Huntington's disease are likely to develop frontotemporal dementia. These people initially have sub-cortical changes related to their movement problems. Because there are many linkages between the sub-cortex and the frontal lobe, the frontal lobe also gets damaged.

Genetics

In about half the cases of frontotemporal dementia there is a family history of similar problems. Some of the inherited forms are related to abnormalities on chromosomes 3 and 17.

What happens in the brain?

In Pick's disease, there is severe shrinkage of the frontal lobes and part of the temporal lobes. In progressive aphasia, it is mainly the left frontal and temporal lobes that are affected. In semantic dementia, the front of the temporal lobes is severely affected.

In Pick's disease, the brain can become full of holes, like a sponge. The nerve cells balloon out and contain large, irregular 'Pick bodies', which can be recognised under the microscope. There is a lot of scarring. The proteins tau and ubiquitin, which are present in Alzheimer's disease, can also be found in Pick's disease. The familial frontotemporal dementias, progressive aphasia and semantic dementia may show brain degradation similar to that seen in Pick's disease, or there may be tiny holes only visible under the microscope. There can also be plaques, tangles and amyloid deposits in the brain cells and around the blood vessels.

Unlike other dementias, there does not appear to be a marked reduction in the levels of acetylcholine or butrylcholine, at least initially.

What tests are available for frontotemporal dementia?

Usually, a specialist makes a diagnosis based on the patient's history, an examination and a number of other tests. The examination may reveal abnormal reflexes, or slowness and stiffness in the familial form of the disease. Doctors look for other signs that suggest the cause of the frontal lobe dementia, such as the abnormal movements in Huntington's disease or signs of alcohol excess. CT or MRI scans may show shrinkage of the frontal or temporal lobes. Psychological testing will show that the frontal lobes are more affected than other areas of the brain.

Can frontotemporal dementia be prevented?

We do not know how to avoid developing frontotemporal dementia. Keeping alcohol intake within moderate limits and avoiding participation in activities that might cause brain injury (such as boxing) will protect the frontal and temporal lobes, to a degree. Following a healthy lifestyle generally might help prevent frontal damage secondary to Alzheimer's disease and vascular dementia.

Alcohol-related dementia

Alcohol is cheap and freely available in New Zealand and many of us have more than the recommended intake of 14 standard drinks per week for women and 21 for men. Alcohol is a 'neurotoxin' that destroys nerve cells. Enough of it, especially with a diet deficient in thiamine (Vitamin B), can result in alcohol-induced persisting dementia. This involves poor short-term memory and impaired frontal lobe function. Unlike the other dementias, there can be an improvement if the person stops drinking — which, of course, is the main challenge.

In summary

Knowing the type of dementia a person has allows us to understand better what is happening and what we might expect. In the next chapters, we look at the course over time of the various kinds of dementia.

Chapter 3

Diagnosis

It is very scary to be diagnosed with an incurable dementing disease. Try to imagine it — you are faced with the knowledge that you are going to lose all your normal mental functions over a period of years, and no one can tell you exactly what will happen when, nor how long it will take.

CHRISTINE BODEN [1]

Sometimes it is difficult to decide whether the forgetfulness exhibited by an older person is normal for someone of their age or whether it is the beginning of dementia. However, when memory loss begins to affect daily life, there is cause for concern. Sometimes a person may give up doing something, like being the secretary to a club or managing the household finances, with only a vague explanation for why they are stopping. The chore is taken on by someone else, who thinks that the person is understandably tired of doing the things they have done all their life. In fact, the person may have been struggling to perform the task because of cognitive (thinking) difficulties.

He was a builder and he probably had Alzheimer's when he was building because he stopped doing his work and used to say there was no work out there, and he said he was depressed . . . and he would make excuses that he couldn't do his carpentry and then he did painting for a while . . .

J. TALKING ABOUT HER HUSBAND WHEN HE WAS IN THE EARLY STAGES OF ALZHEIMER'S DISEASE

At this point, the person may be aware that things are not right. This sense that there is something wrong causes anxiety in most people, and may be accompanied by irritability or loss of confidence. The person may become depressed.

Over time it becomes clear that there are other problems, such as trouble with depth perception or difficulty finding words (not just people's names). Once symptoms like these appear, a diagnosis of dementia can be made. But before that, the memory loss seems just a bit worse than that of other people of the same age and this leaves everyone uncertain about what is happening. To confuse things further, many other things can look like dementia.

Some people doubt the wisdom of even trying to make a diagnosis of dementia. 'There's nothing you can do about it, so why upset the person?' They think it is better for the person to go along in ignorance until the condition has developed to a point where they don't know that there is anything wrong with them, rather than alerting them to the future.

Even before we had drugs to treat dementia, there were problems with this approach. Firstly, a person's memory loss might be caused by something other than dementia, which, if treated, would return the person to mental clarity. Secondly, even if it does turn out that a person has dementia, the person can plan for the future by making important legal or financial decisions and writing advance directives for their care. Now, there is also evidence that the sooner treatment with anti-dementia drugs is begun, the better the chance of maintaining someone at a good level of functioning.

Getting help

It is not usually the person with dementia who decides there is something wrong and seeks help. It is almost always a concerned family member or other close contact.

It is difficult to raise the topic of someone else's failing memory. People are likely to feel angry or hurt if someone questions their mental ability. They may adamantly deny that anything is wrong. In this situation, confronting them usually makes the denial worse. It is probably better to remain sympathetic and alert for an opportunity to introduce the subject again. If the situation becomes dangerous, though, it might be necessary to be more direct.

Sometimes a partner will minimise their spouse's difficulties and gradually, making various excuses, take over their chores. Older men often become much more involved in the domestic routine once they have retired. The man's wife may be eventually left doing very little. It may not be obvious to either party that this situation has occurred because the woman is no longer capable of doing anything, rather than because she has voluntarily let her husband take over. The man who cannot bear to face up to the changes in his beloved wife will angrily reject suggestions from others that she is not well. This can be enormously frustrating to other family members who realise there is something wrong.

Sometimes a parent will take notice of one child but not another. In this situation the favoured family sibling may be able to persuade their parent to see the doctor. It is important to get all the family involved, though, as it may convince the person both of the need to seek help, and also that there is support around if the worst is confirmed.

Most older people have to visit the doctor sooner or later for a repeat prescription or a driving licence medical examination. There is nothing wrong with a concerned family member phoning up beforehand and letting the GP or the practice nurse know of their worries. Although honesty is usually the best policy, on some occasions the older person will be so angry with the person who talks to the doctor that their relationship will be damaged. If this might be the case, tell the surgery that you do not want the person to know you have spoken to them. The doctor can then bring up the subject of memory without implicating the informant. Not every GP wants to do this, but most will understand the difficulties. There is no problem under the Privacy Act in sharing your concerns with the doctor or nurse.

Finally, perhaps if a person knows that dementia is not as hopeless a diagnosis as it once was and that treatment has changed dramatically over recent years, he or she might be willing to be checked out.

Assessment for dementia

GPs do not usually set aside adequate time in an appointment to make a full assessment of a person who may have dementia. You can ask for a long appointment but you may have to pay extra for this. It is very helpful if the concerned person as well as the person with memory loss attends.

The doctor's task is:

1. To confirm that there is evidence of memory or other cognitive impairment.
2. If there is, to investigate *why* the person has this impairment.
3. If there is no obvious problem at this point, the doctor might still need to consider what is going on. Why are people concerned? Does the memory problem fluctuate, or is there another problem, such as deafness or mental illness, which could have led to a confusing picture?

Some GPs are not very interested or expert in the diagnosis of dementia and may refer the person to another service relatively quickly. Others will do a lot of the investigation themselves. Whatever happens, don't be fobbed off with the phrase, 'it's just old age'. It might be, but it is important to check first that it is not any of the alternatives.

Regardless of who makes the assessment, it is likely to include some of the following: patient's history, an examination, blood tests, X-rays, scans and neuro-psychological testing.

History

In this part of the consultation the doctor hears the story of what has happened and asks questions to help clarify the diagnosis. It is helpful if the patient or accompanying person writes down their concerns, as things often get forgotten, especially if people are anxious about the situation. These are the sorts of areas a doctor might consider while taking a patient's history:

What is the main problem? When did it start? How did it start? What did anyone first notice? How have things developed? Has deterioration been gradual or abrupt? Are there additional problems now (like a change in mood or behaviour)? Is there anything that makes it better? Or worse? Has it interfered with the patient's life? How? Are there any recent changes that may have caused the problem; for example, shifting house or a death in the family.

Are there any other symptoms that haven't been mentioned? The doctor might then ask specifically about symptoms of depression, anxiety or delirium (see below).

Past history: Have there been problems like this before? Did they get better spontaneously or did the person receive some treatment? If so, what sort of treatment? Has the person been depressed, anxious or delirious in the past?

Medical history: Does the patient have a medical condition (like diabetes, high blood pressure, high cholesterol, previous strokes, heart problems, head injury, Parkinson's disease) that might be a cause of the problem? Are they suffering from symptoms now that suggest something acute is going on (pain, fever, cough etc.)?

Medication: What drugs is the patient on? Are they being taken as prescribed? (This is an important question as people with memory problems forget vital medicines, or sometimes take them too often.) Are over-the-counter or homeopathic remedies being taken?

Alcohol, cigarettes and other drugs: Does the patient smoke? If yes, how frequently? What is their usual alcohol intake? Has it increased recently? What about other non-prescription drugs (including herbal remedies)?

Family history: Are there any illnesses that run in the family that might now be showing up in this person (Alzheimer's disease, strokes, Huntington's disease) or might indicate a possible predisposition to dementia (Down's syndrome)?

Social situation: Are they managing to keep themselves clean, fed, warm and safe? Can they manage their finances? Who is there to support the person?

Usual personality: Has this changed? Is the person behaving in an unusual fashion?

As an adjunct the doctor (or nurse) might include a questionnaire for the accompanying person, such as the 'Informant Questionnaire on Cognitive Decline in the Elderly' (IQCODE). This is either 16 or 26 questions which take 10–15 minutes to complete. The higher the score, the greater the cognitive decline. Questionnaires can be found at www.crahw.anu.edu.au/files/English_long.pdf and www.crahw.anu.edu.au/files/English_short.pdf.

Examination

This comprises two parts, the physical examination and the mental status examination. Both can be carried out simultaneously — the doctor can observe the person's behaviour, ability to tell their story, answer questions and respond to requests while talking together and during a general physical exam as well as just in conversation.

In the physical exam, the doctor checks especially for heart, blood vessel and blood pressure problems and abnormalities of the nervous system. In the mental state examination the doctor looks for depression or delirium as well as signs of dementia.

A more formal part of the mental status examination is the testing of cognitive function. The doctor asks the patient a standard set of questions, which check the person's ability to remember and think. A commonly used test is the MSQ (below).

MENTAL STATUS QUESTIONNAIRE (MSQ)

1. *What is your age?*
2. *What is the time? (The patient may consult their watch.)*
3. *Repeat this address (the doctor gives patient a random address, e.g. 201 Queen Street. Patient will be required to recall it again at the end of the MSQ).*
4. *What year is it?*
5. *What is the name of this hospital? (Or, what is your home address?)*
6. *Can you name two of the people present in this room? (Patient usually knows doctor and person who has accompanied them to the clinic, e.g. their partner or child.)*
7. *What is your date of birth (only day and month required)?*
8. *What years was the First World War fought?*

> 9. *What is the name of the present Prime Minister?*
> 10. *Count backwards from 20 to 1. (After doing this patient is asked to recall the address given in question 3.)*
>
> *A normal score on the MSQ is 10 out of 10. Any score below 8 is abnormal. A score of 8 or 9 is borderline.*

An alternative is the GPCOG (www.gpcog.com.au). This is a six-question test done in conjunction with a brief informant questionnaire.

The MMSE is a more comprehensive examination which has been widely used internationally. However, recent changes in copyright mean that clinicians are changing to other tools, such as The Montreal Cognitive Assessment (www.mocatest.org). This test measures:

- Visiospatial/executive function
- Naming
- Memory
- Attention
- Language
- Abstraction
- Delayed Recall
- Orientation.

A normal score is 25–30, mild cognitive impairment is 19–25 and dementia is diagnosed at 11–21. (Note the overlap of mild cognitive impairment with dementia — if function is affected, a dementia diagnosis is made.)

With the loss of the MMSE, various other tests are also in use. Generally they cover the sorts of fields listed above. Tests can be affected by language, educational level, anxiety, tiredness, poor hearing and a host of other factors. Because tests involve writing, reading and drawing, poor vision (even being without your reading glasses) and physical problems (such as a stroke or Parkinson's disease) can affect them.

These tests are only rough guides that indicate that something *might* be going on. Getting a low score does not necessarily mean that the person has dementia, but it does require an explanation. The explanation could be anything from the fact that the person has had a lifelong intellectual disability to the person being too depressed to try to answer the questions, or a whole host of other factors.

The pattern of the results can help indicate what is going on. In Alzheimer's disease the person might not be orientated and would do poorly on memory and naming objects. In Lewy body dementia, visiospatial skills and attention are affected early. If a person is depressed, he or she sometimes just answers, 'I don't know'. In Parkinson's disease the responses might be accurate, but very slow.

Blood tests

There is no blood test that shows whether or not a person has dementia. However, blood tests can show whether there is anything wrong which could make a person confused or make memory loss worse.

The usual tests are:

- Thyroid function (an over- or underactive thyroid will affect thinking)
- Vitamin B12 (lack of this vitamin can cause memory problems) and folate levels
- Calcium levels (a high calcium level can cause confusion)
- Full blood count (looks for anaemia or evidence of infection)
- Electrolyte levels (low sodium can cause confusion, other abnormalities indicate poor health)
- Urea and/or creatinine levels (these measure kidney function: if it is abnormal it can cause confusion and might be the cause of any electrolyte imbalance)
- Homocysteine levels: a high level indicates vascular disease and may also be relevant to Alzheimer's disease
- Other tests: These are done if the doctor thinks they might be relevant; for example, tests for syphilis (rare now, but once a major cause of dementia). AIDS can cause dementia and so, if the person is at risk, an HIV test is needed. While the person is having a blood test, the doctor might also check out their blood glucose and lipids (including cholesterol). It is important to know these levels if a vascular dementia is suspected.

X-rays and scans

Sometimes the doctor will order a chest X-ray if there could be something wrong with the heart or lungs which could interfere with the supply of oxygen to the brain. Generally, however, this is not necessary.

CT or CAT scan: This stands for 'computerised (axial) tomography' and is a series of pictures taken in slices across (axial) the brain. Put together, they form a three-dimensional representation of the brain. The expert radiologist who reads the scan can recognise changes in tone, structure and volume of different parts of the brain. These changes enable the radiologist to diagnose brain tumours, strokes or other injuries and hydrocephalus (increased fluid around the brain) among other things. In the early stages of Alzheimer's disease the brain may appear normal or show only the shrinkage that would be expected due to age. Measurements of the hippocampus can help decide whether the patient has developed Alzheimer's disease (though not all radiologists are trained in this).

MRI scan: This stands for 'magnetic resonance imaging' and takes finer pictures of the brain and is particularly good at picking up tiny strokes or other changes related to poor blood supply. It is useful for assessing vascular dementia.

If the patient has signs and symptoms typical of Alzheimer's disease and there are no abnormal findings on examination, a scan is not particularly useful. However, if there is anything unusual about the examination or history, for example, rapid onset or a known head injury, then a scan can be helpful.

The scan can be performed either privately or in the public system. A private CT scan costs about $350 and can sometimes be claimed back on medical insurance, depending on the type of policy (check this out first). In the public system there is usually a waiting time, but this varies around the country depending on the local situation and the degree of urgency indicated by the doctor when asking for a scan.

For a CT scan, the person has to lie in a tube-like structure and hold his or her head relatively still for about five minutes. People who find the experience frighteningly claustrophobic can take medication to calm them during the test. An MRI scan is noisy, and this often bothers people. It also takes much longer than a CT scan (up to 30 minutes). Sometimes, the radiologist will inject a dye (contrast) into a vein in order to make the picture clearer. People who are allergic to iodine, which is in the dye, need to let the radiologist know this.

SPECT (Single Photon Emission Computerised Tomography) and PET (Positron Emission Tomography) scans: can show changes in the *function* (not just the structure) of the brain. These are mainly used in research, although very occasionally may help with diagnosis if the symptoms are unusual.

Neuropsychological testing

A psychologist will carry out a series of question-and-answer type tests to sort out what is happening to the patient. These tests can be very helpful in diagnosing difficult cases; for example, distinguishing depression from dementia, and determining exactly which part of the brain is involved and how much. The tests involve questions similar to those in the MMSE or MOCA, but far more detailed, as well as various pen and paper tests and puzzles.

Some people quite enjoy them. The tests can be tiring, though, taking between 45 minutes and several hours. They are expensive because they involve a lot of time with a highly trained specialist and, as a result, are performed only occasionally. They are usually done through the public hospital system, though in some areas are available (at some cost) in the private system. As well as being useful for diagnosis, the tests can identify areas of strength and weakness, which helps carers understand the person better and may help therapists develop ways round their patient's difficulties.

What looks like dementia but isn't?

Many things other than dementia can affect memory and thinking. In the older age group, common problems that can cause dementia-like symptoms are:

- Delirium (acute confusion)
- Depression
- Medication side effects
- Excess alcohol
- Head injury
- Brain disorders other than dementia
- Other medical problems.

People with poor vision or hearing may not take things in and so can appear to have forgotten them. However, their memories are fine, once they have registered the relevant information. Someone with intellectual disability might appear to have dementia the first time you meet them. However, people who have known them over a long period of time can confirm that there is no change in memory or other function.

It is possible that a doctor will discover some sort of illness or abnormality that needs to be sorted out before they can tell whether the main problem is dementia. Delirium, depression and drug side effects are the most common conditions that can be confused with dementia.

Delirium (acute confusion)

These are the symptoms of delirium:

SIGNS AND SYMPTOMS OF DELIRIUM (DSM IV)[2]

- *Disturbance in level of consciousness (reduced clarity of awareness of the environment)*
- *A change in cognition (such as memory, orientation, language disturbance) or the development of a perceptual problem (usually hallucinations — seeing or hearing things that are not there)*
- *The disturbance develops over a short period of time (hours to days) and tends to fluctuate over the course of a day*
- *Evidence from history and examination that there is something medically wrong.*

Delirium compared with dementia

Characteristically delirium comes on suddenly. It is not the slow, gradual process that occurs in Alzheimer's disease, Lewy body dementia or frontal lobe dementia. However, vascular dementia can show sudden changes and a small stroke may cause delirium.

The person with delirium has a variable level of alertness. He or she might be completely lucid at one moment and drowsy or very confused at another. A delirious person can be very frightened and restless or even aggressive, or may sit in an abnormally quiet way, only occasionally rousing. This change in the level of alertness is rare in Alzheimer's disease, vascular dementia or the frontotemporal dementias. Visual hallucinations (seeing things that are not there) often occur in delirium, but less commonly in dementia, other than the Lewy body type. Lewy body dementia is difficult to distinguish from delirium because in both there are fluctuations in alertness and often hallucinations.

Delirium can be caused by many medical conditions. Commonly, infections, medications, chemical imbalances, heart attack or strokes are the problem, but there are many more causes. Once the underlying condition is treated, the delirium gradually abates. This can take weeks to months in older people and the recovery is not always complete. People with an underlying dementia are more prone to becoming delirious. It is not always easy to decide what is happening when presented with a case of delirium.

Depression

This common psychiatric illness can look like dementia. Depression is a distressing condition but treatment will help the person think more clearly again.

SIGNS AND SYMPTOMS OF DEPRESSION (DSM IV) [3]

- *Low mood or lack of emotions*
- *Loss of interest and pleasure*
- *Changed sleep pattern (often insomnia)*
- *Change in appetite (usually reduced)*
- *Poor concentration or memory*
- *Increased anxiety or irritability*
- *Agitation, i.e. increased meaningless activity (like pacing), or slowing down*
- *Guilty thoughts, feelings of hopelessness*
- *Recurrent thoughts of death or suicide.*

Some people with depression develop delusions (false beliefs), for example, that they are very poor or have a dreadful disease. Some may have hallucinations, especially auditory hallucinations, sometimes hearing voices telling them that they are a bad person.

Some of the symptoms of depression could be easily mistaken for dementia. Loss of interest in life might mean that a woman stops caring properly for herself. Poor concentration could stop a man from paying the bills as usual. People often complain of a poor memory when they are depressed, because they cannot take things in. Depressed people may focus on all the things they have done wrong, and so will not remember where they left their keys or that they were meant to be at an appointment. People with depression often believe that they are 'losing their mind' and it might appear this way to others too.

It is often difficult, even for a doctor, to differentiate between depression and dementia. If this is the case, it is worth treating the patient for depression, even if the diagnosis is not entirely clear. Standard treatment uses drugs or psychotherapy, or both. It usually takes eight to twelve weeks to see the full effects of treatment, and it is important to be patient. Antidepressants are not addictive and the newer types do not have too many side effects.

Medication side effects

Many older people are on a large number of drugs for different medical conditions. The table contains a list of drugs that might either cause confusion or make it worse.

DRUGS THAT CAUSE OR WORSEN CONFUSION [4]

- *Drugs for treatment of mental disorders: antidepressants: usually the older type, such as amitriptyline, lithium, sedatives, Valium-type medication and sleeping pills; major tranquillisers: drugs used for psychotic symptoms, such as chlorpromazine, thioridazine and some of the newer sorts like risperidone*
- *Recreational drugs: alcohol and others*
- *Painkillers and anti-inflammatory drugs: steroids, such as prednisone, Digesic, morphine-like drugs and drugs like naproxen (Naprosyn), diclofenac (Voltaren) and celec oxib (Celebrex). (Paracetamol is OK.)*
- *Anticholinergic drugs: drugs used for bladder control, such as Ditropan, drugs for bowel cramps or diarrhoea (for example, Buscopan), over-the-counter remedies for coughs and colds*
- *Anticonvulsants: drugs used for epilepsy, especially if they sedate people*
- *Antidiabetic drugs: for example, glibenclamide or metformin, if they cause low blood sugar*
- *Antihistamines used for allergies or in flu and cold treatments*
- *Parkinson's drugs: for example, Sinemet, bromocriptine*
- *Heart or blood pressure drugs: beta-blockers or digoxin*
- *Miscellaneous: ciprofloxacin (an antibiotic), quinine (for cramps), theophylline (to aid breathing), H-2 antagonists (for stomach troubles including ulcers).*

If the person does not need the offending drug, their doctor can stop their medication to see if the confusion abates. It is usually not this easy, though, as the person's condition may necessitate the medication prescribed. It may be possible to reduce the dose or replace the medication with another drug, which does the same job without causing confusion. Changes in medication need to be done slowly and carefully. As with all treatments, a balance between good and bad effects needs to be found, and the outcome may not be perfect.

Who makes the diagnosis?

Often general practitioners are uncomfortable about making the diagnosis of such a serious condition as dementia without a specialist's opinion. They may refer someone with memory loss to another doctor with more expertise in this area. The patient or the family can ask for another opinion as well as the GP's, if this is what they want.

Specialists with an interest and training in the diagnosis and treatment of dementia are:

Neurologists: physicians with special training in disorders of the brain and nervous system.
Psychiatrists: doctors who deal with mental illness.
Geriatricians: physicians working with older people.
Psychogeriatricians: psychiatrists with a special interest in mental illness in older people.

Memory clinics: In many areas there are specialised clinics (usually run by geriatricians or psychogeriatricians) that deal specifically with memory problems. Check with your GP or local hospital to see if there is one in your district.

Neurologists are skilled at making diagnoses. They are especially good at sorting out the unusual causes of memory loss and tend to deal with younger people with such difficulties. They are less involved in the ongoing care of people with dementia or very elderly people with multiple problems. Neurologists work in both the private or public sectors. They are very much in demand, and there is often a long wait to see them in either system. Medical insurance that covers specialists' fees will pay for a neurologist (at least partially). Check the cost when phoning up for a private appointment. In the public system, the patient attends a clinic in the local hospital, where, as well as seeing a doctor, the various other tests can be carried out.

Psychiatrists see people who have psychological or behavioural difficulties as well as memory loss. They can distinguish between dementia and other mental disorders, such as depression. Most psychogeriatricians work in teams in the public sector. Often a nurse from the team will do the first assessment in the person's home and the psychogeriatrician will see the person later, either at home or as an outpatient at the hospital.

There are a few psychogeriatricians working in private practice. The patient would be seen in the specialist's rooms or at home. The cost of an assessment may be covered by insurance.

Geriatricians are experts at distinguishing medical problems from dementia. They can then treat the medical problems and/or arrange community services to help the person with failing cognitive abilities. They, or members of their teams, visit people at home or see them in an outpatient clinic. Geriatricians almost always work in the public system, but sometimes do a little part-time private practice. Your local GP can find out about this. Waiting lists are not usually very long in the public or private systems.

All three types of specialist can admit people to hospital, but this is rarely necessary at the assessment stage.

What if you still don't know?

Even after all the tests, second opinions and treatments, it may still not be possible to confirm a diagnosis of dementia. If this is the case, the doctor will usually reassess the patient in six months' time to check for changes that suggest a decline in cognition. It is very hard to wait around for months with this uncertainty. However, people usually have their own ways of managing in these circumstances. Some like to get as much information as they can about dementia to be prepared for the worst. Others just put the worry to the back of their minds and get on with life as best they can. Some people complete preparations for an uncertain future, such as appointing a power of attorney or writing their memoirs.

Whatever the outcome, dementia is no longer a sentence that commits you to losing your mind and your dignity or being locked up in a humiliating institution. The good news is that things are changing for the better.

References

[1] Boden, Christine, *Who Will I Be When I Die?* HarperCollins, Sydney, 1997, p. 54.

[2] *Diagnostic and Statistical Manual of Psychiatric Disorders*, 4th edition, The American Psychiatric Association, Washington, 1994.

[3] Ibid.

[4] National Advisory Committee on Health and Disability/ADARDS, *Guidelines for the Support and Management of People with Dementia*, Ministry of Health, Wellington, 1997.

Chapter 4

Early-stage dementia

I feel that I am slowly becoming
'uncertain', I forget things, times, people
I am not sure what I should do.
I discovered a place where I could buy
things . . . but have forgotten where it is.
I am afraid to go ahead and do things.
As I write at the window I am not sure
where the road, left or write [sic] goes. Opposite
to me is a man who has sat opposite me
for many, many times . . . but I don't know
his name, I think it is Sunday, I am
not sure if I should go to church.
I think Alison is coming after lunch
to take me to their house — There are
children at the house: I know them but
I am not sure what they will be doing.
'Uncertainty' is not the same as 'madness'
but it is groying [sic] that way. I can talk
about things & people but it is very
much a cover-up, and I don't follow it up.[1]

The poem above was found among a gentleman's possessions when his home was cleared out after he had been admitted into residential care. It graphically illustrates the feelings and thoughts of a person in early-stage dementia. Mild or early dementia is defined as that stage when people, although they have been diagnosed as having dementia, can still manage their daily lives. They require little assistance from others.

Telling the person

Once a diagnosis of dementia has been made, the first decision is what to tell the person. Should you tell a person that they have dementia? This topic has been hotly debated for years.

One of the main complaints from families of people with dementia is that they were not given enough information about their relative's condition.

Studies of these families show that although they want to know the diagnosis, many of them do not think the person should be told. They fear the person with dementia will get anxious or depressed once they know the diagnosis. At the same time they almost all say that if it were them who had the disorder, they would want to know. About half the families who had thought it was a good idea to tell people they have dementia said that informing the person of the diagnosis had been harmful. The picture is confusing if you talk to families, but even professionals are not at all clear about what to do. Doctors often find it hard to make a diagnosis of dementia, and they do not wish to unduly frighten people by giving them wrong news.

If there was nothing that could be done about dementia, then it might be reasonable to spare the person with dementia the truth, knowing that, in time, the person would lose any awareness that there was something wrong. However, there are decisions that need to be made while the person is still capable of doing so. These include making plans for future care, for example, where to live, whether to have treatment for certain conditions and how to manage finances. There is also the decision about whether to take medication that might slow the progress of the disorder. The person with dementia may also want to take the opportunity to talk through things with their family, and there is a grieving process for all to go through. Finally, keeping an illness secret from the person and others tends to reinforce the stigma surrounding it.

On the other hand, neither families nor professionals have the right to impose their own values on a person with dementia. Some people make it clear that they don't want to be told their diagnosis. The question that then arises is whether people are entitled not to know, if that is their choice.

There is no one right answer. During the process of assessment, the doctor may get a sense of how much or little the patient wants to know. If the patient is kept up to date with the results of the assessment, then the diagnosis will not come as such a shock. It also gives the person with dementia the chance to say, 'Don't tell me about it, but let my son know . . .' if that is what they want.

Most people will want to know the diagnosis at some point, and the necessary information can be given gradually and sensitively, in as much detail as the person seems to want. The person with dementia needs to be reassured at every opportunity that they won't be abandoned and that there will always be someone there to care for them. New medications offer hope for slowing or even temporarily arresting the progress of the disease.

People remember very little about interviews when they are told devastating news (even if their brains are perfectly normal), so it might be useful for the patient or their family to ask for a brief written summary of what has been discussed. (Some doctors provide a tape recording of the consultation.) The diagnosing doctor should be available for discussion later when the person or family wants clarification or repetition of information.

If the doctor misreads the patient and gives them too much information, then denial or forgetfulness may protect the person from the full emotional impact of this unwanted information. As in any other life-threatening illness, a person who receives such traumatic news may go into a state of shock or disbelief. Later they may become angry, guilty or depressed.

Who else should be told?

People with recently diagnosed dementia can decide whom they would like told about their condition. If they choose not to say anything to anyone, that is their decision. Only when patients put themselves or others in danger can their doctor inform others against the patient's wishes. If the person is not capable of making decisions (see chapter 17) then the doctor should inform the next-of-kin or caregiver. Mostly, people want to share the bad news with someone else, but there are some very private people who do not want anyone to know what is happening. This wish has to be respected, however uncomfortable the health professional feels about it.

It is hard to predict the reactions of older friends to the diagnosis of dementia. Sometimes it helps to explain puzzling behaviour and comes as a relief. Sometimes people respond by staying away, as if the disorder were contagious. Many older people are anxious around people who have developed something that they themselves fear. Different cultural groups have different responses, varying from shame and rejection to openness and acceptance, and this will affect who is told. In recent years, famous people such as Ronald Reagan, Iris Murdoch and Terry Pratchett have publicly acknowledged having Alzheimer's disease. Hopefully, this new openness will help reduce the fear and stigma surrounding dementia.

What if people don't believe there is anything wrong?

A common response to the development of dementia is to deny that there is anything wrong. This could be a 'psychological defence' — that is, an unconscious mental process working to protect people from devastating knowledge — or it could be the result of actual brain damage (especially to the frontal lobe) so that people lose the ability to appreciate changes in themselves. This refusal (or inability) to accept that there is something wrong means that a person can reject offers of help and neglect making plans for the future. The denial can be partial:

> *Yes, my memory is not so good, but I don't need to do anything about it just yet . . .*

or complete:

> *There's nothing wrong with me . . . I'm managing fine!*

There is not a lot that others can do about a person who denies their cognitive powers are failing. If they insist that the person faces up to reality, they may get an angry response and ruin their relationship. The denial is there for a purpose, and if it is broken down the person could be overwhelmed by terror or despair. If there are tasks that must be done, it is better to get around this by an indirect approach. For example, a lawyer with their client could discuss the usefulness of an Enduring Power of Attorney without reference to that person's current illness.

A spouse also sometimes goes into denial, protecting both themself and their partner from the knowledge of what is happening.

> *The husband at the medical assessment says laughingly, 'Well, my memory is pretty bad too . . .'*

This might mean that the partner refuses to accept help or discourages the person with dementia from receiving appropriate care. A professional or family member should not collude by agreeing that there is nothing wrong, but needs to try to understand why the person is unable to accept the truth. The husband may be terrified that his lifetime partner will be removed from his care and company, or that he will lose control of the situation in other ways. He might think that bossy children or professionals will tell him how to look after his beloved wife of many decades. He may feel that her situation is somehow of his making — perhaps he didn't care for her well enough in their earlier life, and he needs to make up for this. Or, more simply, caring for his wife gives him meaning in life and he fears that this will be taken away. These worries may have to be gently addressed, to allow him to acknowledge her disability and permit additional support as necessary.

It may help, in cases like this, to point out that the husband will be able to continue giving care longer if he has some help. He can be reassured that he will continue to have input into what happens to his wife. If he is the sole elderly caregiver, the big worry is that he will become suddenly ill and be unable to provide care. For everyone's peace of mind, there needs to be discussion about alternative arrangements for emergencies.

Children accept the reality of a parent's dementia at different rates. This can be the cause of very upsetting conflict. One person (usually the one who has most to do with the parent) will become aware of the problems sooner than more distant relatives. These distant relatives may accuse the close one of making a fuss about nothing or make out that things are not all that bad. This is especially likely if the person is seen only at family gatherings, spruced up for the occasion, and still able to engage in social conversation. On the other hand, it is sometimes easier for family who see their parents only occasionally to notice changes than for those who see them on a daily basis.

Sometimes a husband or wife is very aware that their spouse is not well, but their children deny there is anything wrong. This can be a problem if the marital relationship has been difficult, or the family have taken sides with one parent or the other. The children of a first marriage may be reluctant to hear the pleas of their stepmother who is struggling with their father.

One way of reinforcing the message is for the caregiver to get the doubters to spend some time with the person with dementia. They may then (grudgingly) acknowledge that things are as the carer reported.

Early changes

The different types of dementia progress in their own fashion. As the course of Alzheimer's disease is the best studied and most predictable, I will describe Alzheimer's first, but note the differences for other forms of dementia. There are common themes, and as the dementias advance they begin to look alike.

These changes can be very distressing for the person with dementia but, with the progress of the illness, many people lose awareness that there is something wrong and seem to suffer less. For their family, whanau and friends, though, it can be very painful to watch the long, slow, occasionally alarming deterioration of someone they love. Some people want to know what is going to happen to them as the disease progresses. This gives them a sense of control. Others prefer to take one day at a time, dealing with problems as they arise. This may help to maintain hope.

Alzheimer's disease

Short-term memory loss

Early in Alzheimer's disease a person will have difficulties with short-term memory. Short-term memory is memory for recent events: what the person did yesterday, where she put her handbag, what he did with his wallet, what has been planned for the day's activities. This forgetfulness is probably what called attention to the fact that something is wrong and led to the medical investigation and diagnosis. The person's long-term memory, on the other hand, is undamaged and there may be excellent recall of earlier life.

Such memory loss can be extremely frustrating, both to the person with dementia and the people around them. Common problems resulting from short-term memory loss are:

- Repetition of questions, as the person has forgotten the answer
- Difficulty following conversations and contributing only superficial, social comments or questions; for example, repeating 'How are you?' or 'What are your children doing now?' despite these questions having already been answered
- Being unable to follow what is happening on TV
- Not being able to learn new things or follow instructions
- Trouble using the telephone because the person can't remember the numbers or how to put them in the right order
- Losing things, especially when put in new places to 'keep them safe'.

Poor sense of direction

Loss of sense of direction, especially in a new place, occurs fairly early on in Alzheimer's. Sometimes this is the thing that really brings the person's dementia to their attention, occasionally in an alarming way as in the example below.

> *Mrs K. was terrified when her husband failed to return to their hotel while on holiday in Kuala Lumpur. After three hours of searching between the hotel and the market where she had left him, Mrs K. discovered him, cheerful enough and puzzled by her agitation. The problem was not only his poor sense of direction, but also the fact that he had forgotten he was supposed to meet her back at the hotel. She stuck close to him for the rest of the trip.*

Some people have trouble finding the bathroom in a new place, especially at night, when there are no visual clues to guide them, but are perfectly all right in their own homes.

Executive skills loss

The planning, organising and decision-making skills necessary for managing both work and finances may be lost early on. Some of this may result from poor short-term memory, as well as from the effect of the disease on the frontal lobe. The outcome is that bills are left unpaid and important letters are ignored.

Occasionally a person's dementia only comes to light when the council goes in to turn off their water because of unpaid rates. People sometimes find they are unable to continue their usual line of work — an office worker may not know what to do about the papers on their desk. In professional fields, people with dementia may make decisions that are not in the best interests of their clients or, worse, are dangerous. For the self-employed this loss of ability to work can be financially disastrous:

> *He couldn't write the invoices properly. I had to see to all the money. I had to see to the GST.*
>
> J. TALKING ABOUT HER HUSBAND WITH EARLY ALZHEIMER'S DISEASE

Difficulty concentrating and not being distracted

It is difficult for people with dementia to concentrate on one thing, especially when there are a lot of things happening around them. They need to make a great effort to focus their attention and this leads to tiredness and an exaggeration of other problems. People with dementia may tire easily in social situations and need to withdraw. The family needs to be aware of this so that if the person seems to be getting overwhelmed or confused, they can gently suggest a rest or some time in a quiet place. Robert Davis writes in his book, *My Journey into Alzheimer's Disease*:

> In my present condition [seven months since diagnosis] there are times when I feel normal. At other times I cannot follow what is going on around me; the conversation whips too fast from person to person and before I have processed one comment, the thread has moved to another person or another topic, and I am left isolated from the action . . . alone in a crowd. If I press myself with greatest concentration to try to keep up, I feel as though something short-circuits in my brain. At this point I become disorientated, have difficulty with my balance if I am standing, my speech becomes slow, or I cannot find the right words to express myself.[2]

Emotional changes

There are many emotional changes that may occur in the early stages of dementia.

Increased anxiety: If someone knows something is happening but can't remember what, they can feel very insecure. They may also doubt that their family will want them in this condition and so fear being abandoned. This uncertainty can be tackled by reminders, writing things down and sticking to a routine; the anxiety can be reduced by reassurance and affection from friends and family.

Anger and frustration: Tasks that used to be easy now become difficult and things are always lost. It is infuriating that it is so hard to do anything properly. People with dementia may need to limit their expectations: do one thing at a time, leave plenty of time to do things and be methodical, perhaps writing out the steps to each task in advance.

Suspiciousness: Because people with poor memory misplace things they can come to believe that they have been stolen or that people are playing tricks on them by hiding or removing things. They need to be encouraged to ask others about things that are lost. Chapter 7 contains hints for recalling where items have been left.

Feelings of worthlessness and uselessness: Some people find it so difficult to do things they give up and let others take over. They feel as if they have lost their role in life. However, there will always be things that they can do and they will be able to contribute, although this may be in a different way from before.

Embarrassment in social situations: It becomes so hard to cope with multiple conversations and contacts that some people avoid going out. They then risk becoming isolated and bored. Such people might need to be more selective about where they go, choosing places that aren't too noisy or crowded, or making sure they go with someone who understands their situation and can rescue them if necessary.

Loss of motivation, boredom: People with dementia give up old hobbies or interests, stop taking up new ones and become restless, bored or demanding as a result. However, there will probably be things that they can do. Family, friends or an Alzheimer's support group can help them take an active interest in life.

Depression: Knowing that you have a progressive neurological disorder is depressing. Patients will go through the grief process, and most come to accept the changes that the illness will bring. Counselling or medication can help people through this difficult period.

Many people diagnosed with dementia cope extremely well. They remain reasonably philosophical, just taking one day at a time. If people are not aware of their disorder, they may continue on cheerfully as if nothing had changed.

Changes in function and behaviour

Obviously not everyone undergoes the same changes at the same stage of dementia. However, Barry Reisberg, a psychiatrist in New York, has studied hundreds of people with Alzheimer's disease and developed a guide called Functional Assessment Staging (FAST). This guide allows us to assess what a person might be able to do during the various stages of this progressive illness (see below).[3] It can be disheartening to look at the gradual loss of skills that occurs, but understanding what is happening to someone allows us to adjust our expectations accordingly. For example, if a person with mild dementia loses bladder control, there is likely to be something else wrong with them, perhaps a urine infection, as people with Alzheimer's disease retain bladder control until they are much more severely affected. On the other hand, if someone has mild dementia and is no longer able to competently pay their bills, such an occurrence would be expected. This might be the right point to sensitively offer help.

A rule of thumb in Alzheimer's disease is that skills are lost roughly in the reverse order that they are gained over a lifetime. Complex social skills learned in early adulthood are lost sooner than talking and walking, which are learned as a young child. This rule of thumb does not necessarily apply in other forms of dementia.

EARLY-STAGE DEMENTIA

1. *No difficulty, either subjectively (noticed by the person) or objectively (noticed by anyone else).*
2. *Complains of forgetting location of objects. Subjective work difficulties.*
3. *Deficits noted in demanding occupational and social settings. Decreased organisational capacity.*
4. *Deficits in complex tasks of daily life, e.g. handling personal finances, planning/preparing meals.*
5. *Requires assistance in choosing proper clothing to wear for the day or season, e.g. patient may wear the same clothing repeatedly, unless supervised.*

Functional Assessment Staging (FAST)

Vascular dementia

Cognitive changes

The effects of loss of short-term memory are the same whatever the cause. In vascular dementia, there are likely also to be other neurological problems, and the changes that result from these will depend on which part of the brain has been damaged. These changes could include trouble finding the right word, difficulty recognising objects and putting them to use or losing the ability to calculate. Loss of executive skills may occur earlier than short-term memory loss if the frontal lobes are the part of the brain first affected.

Emotional changes

How people react to these cognitive problems will depend on their personality and the amount and location of the brain damage. Unlike those with Alzheimer's disease, people with vascular dementia are often painfully aware that there is something wrong. This can lead to acute anxiety and depression. The difficulties encountered and the associated frustration make people irritable, which can annoy or frighten others.

People who have had multiple strokes may also become overly emotional (the medical term is 'labile'), laughing or crying at the slightest provocation. There may be abrupt, excessive mood changes; for example, becoming suddenly angry over a minor incident. Sometimes people with vascular dementia respond inappropriately; for example, crying at something funny. This can cause a great deal of distress and embarrassment, especially as people often know that they are displaying the wrong emotion or that their reaction is extreme. Lability often responds to treatment with antidepressants, even though patients are not actually suffering from depression.

Changes in function and behaviour

Changes in function and behaviour depend on the area of the brain affected, and the person's response to the change. A person might have trouble with certain skills, such as dressing, because of loss of awareness of one side of their body or because they've forgotten the movements involved in pulling on a sock. Difficulties with speech occur frequently. If the frontal lobe is involved, the person's behaviour may be similar to that seen in frontal lobe dementia (acting impulsively, exhibiting poor judgement, having difficulties making decisions and so on) and may cause problems in social situations or at work.

Lewy body dementia

Cognitive changes

Because the confusion associated with Lewy body dementia varies from hour to hour and day to day, it is often difficult to make a definite diagnosis. Early on, there may be periods of such clarity that the person appears back to their old self. Later, this may change and the person is again disorientated and unable to function, much to everyone's disappointment.

Typically, sufferers have a poor attention span; that is, they are unable to concentrate on one thing for very long. This makes it hard to do things like balance a chequebook or watch a whole TV programme. Attention difficulties can be revealed with testing by the person's inability to do calculations and to concentrate (for example, on spelling a word backwards).

Early on in Lewy body dementia people may have problems judging distance, recognising patterns or finding their way. These are highlighted by getting patients to copy a diagram. However, in contrast to Alzheimer's disease, the sufferer's short-term memory initially may be good.

Emotional and psychological changes

In the early stages of Lewy body dementia people might have visual hallucinations, which commonly involve seeing people or animals that make no noise. The reaction to these can be anything from intense fear to indifference or even amusement. Depression is frequent, occurring in about 40 per cent of cases; this is more common than in Alzheimer's disease.

Changes in function and behaviour

Often people with Lewy body dementia develop low blood pressure on standing, so they become dizzy or unsteady. Faints or falls may be an early feature of the illness and people may be found mute and barely conscious. Stiffness, shaking, slowing down, shuffling, a stooped posture, and similar symptoms suggestive of Parkinson's disease may occur at any stage of the illness.

Frontal lobe dementia

Cognitive changes

The first changes in frontal lobe dementia are likely to be changes in personality and social behaviour. People may become tactless, just saying what they think regardless of the situation. They may breach the rules of social etiquette, which are all around us, but of which we only become aware when broken: examples include failing to introduce a person, overriding someone speaking, not holding the lift, and pushing in front of others in a queue. The following case describes a usually respectable man making unwanted sexual advances.

Mr G., a retired businessman living in a small town, became obsessed with one of the workers at the Post Office. He would go to the Post Office several times a day and always stand in her queue. He bought her flowers and gifts, which she found very embarrassing. People thought he was just infatuated, but when he started following her home, she called the police.

The policeman who visited realised that there was something wrong with Mr G. and he asked for a mental health assessment. Mr G.'s assessment indicated frontal lobe problems and a CT scan showed that he had had several strokes which had damaged both frontal lobes.

Emotional changes

People with frontotemporal damage may lose the capacity to express emotion or to recognise emotion in other people. They may show an empty sort of cheerfulness and make facetious jokes or tell stories in bad taste. Their 'happiness' seems to be superficial and does not communicate itself to others in the way that genuinely happy feelings often do.

Sometimes the lack of emotional expression, social withdrawal and loss of drive seem like depression. However, the changes in frontal lobe dementia are not accompanied by the other changes that occur in depression, and people with frontal lobe dementia often have no concern about what is happening.

Changes in function and behaviour

Frontotemporal dementia may result in reduced activity — for example, a normally active housewife may spend her day sitting watching TV rather than doing her usual work — or increased activity, which often seems pointless or purposeless to an observer. There may be deterioration in the person's level of hygiene or dressing. A previously smartly dressed woman might go out in her slippers and a food-stained cardigan. This is not because people lose the physical skills to dress or wash (as might occur in vascular dementia), but because they lose motivation and social awareness.

A sudden change in food preferences or taking on a new style of dress could be an early sign of frontal lobe dementia. Of course, people are allowed to start dressing in purple or eating Japanese food as they grow older! These changes need to be taken in context as part of the person's overall behaviour.

Advice

Things to do in the early stages of dementia

Financial and legal

- *Talk to the bank about arranging the finances so that they can be managed by someone else if necessary; for example, putting accounts under joint names.*
- *Discuss management of other financial issues; for example, share portfolio.*
- *Arrange for bills to be paid, perhaps by direct debit.*
- *Make sure your will and insurance policies are in order.*
- *Contact Work and Income New Zealand about benefits.*
- *Appoint an Enduring Power of Attorney for property and welfare (see chapter 17).*
- *Write down preferences for future care, possibly including decisions about life-prolonging treatment.*
- *Make decisions about gifting possessions, heirlooms etc., and write these decisions down.*
- *Write down what should be done with pets later if you cannot look after them.*
- *Complete unfinished business of any kind.*

Educational

Find out what you need to know about the illness from as many sources as you can. The national Alzheimer's information line is 0800 004 001. Your local branch of Alzheimer's New Zealand will be in your phone book and there is a website (www.alzheimers.org.nz). Age Concern may be able to answer specific questions or point you in the right direction for help. (Look in the local phone book for the number.) Eldernet is a New Zealand information service for older people. It is not specifically for people with dementia, but offers information on community groups, home services, retirement villages, and residential care. Their website is www.eldernet.co.nz

Investigate various forms of dementia treatment, their costs and efficacy (see chapters 7 and 8).

Getting support

- Tell friends and family as desired. Ask them to help out as needed. Talk to people who have come to terms with having dementia themselves or are caring for an affected relative.
- Attend courses or join a group at your local Alzheimer's New Zealand branch.
- Contact DASN (the Dementia Advocacy and Support Network); their website is www.dasninternational.org

Maximise your abilities

- Work hard to maintain as many skills as possible. Don't let the family take over things you can still do.
- Arrange your home and other aspects of your life to make tasks simpler; for example, remove unnecessary clutter and develop a system of reminders.
- Make sure your physical health is as good as it can be. Get your sight and hearing tested, and teeth attended to.
- Develop a regular exercise programme (see your doctor first).

In summary

Once people have come to terms with the diagnosis, the early stages of dementia can be a relatively peaceful time; a time for people with dementia and their families to enjoy each other. They need to make plans and investigate support services for the future and adjust their expectations of life. The next chapter looks at the moderate stage of dementia.

References

[1] Goldsmith, Malcolm, *Hearing the Voices of People with Dementia: Opportunities and obstacles*, Jessica Kingsley Publishers, London, 1996, pp. 159–60.

[2] Davis, Robert, *My Journey into Alzheimer's Disease*, Tyndale House Publishers, Wheaton, Illinois, 1989, pp. 96–7.

[3] Reisberg, Barry, 'Functional Assessment Staging (FAST)', *Geriatrics,* 41:30–46, 1986.

Chapter 5

Moderate dementia

I do not ask to walk smooth paths
Nor bear an easy load
I pray for strength and fortitude
To climb the rock strewn road.

EMILY BRONTË

Dementia progresses at a variable rate, depending on the underlying cause and the treatment available. The severity of the disorder is measured by the amount it has affected a person's ability to function. Dementia is regarded as moderate when people cannot manage by themselves and need assistance. This chapter covers moderate Alzheimer's disease, then addresses differences in other forms of dementia.

Alzheimer's disease

About four to seven years after the first onset of symptoms (often sooner in young people) the severity of the Alzheimer's disease is likely to progress to the 'moderate' stage. Speech deteriorates and people have to communicate in other ways. This can be frustrating both for people with dementia and their families alike.

As people become less able to function normally, and are perhaps unsafe, carers have to take over various tasks. However, it is really important for the self-esteem of people with dementia that they maintain their skills and independence for as long as possible. One of the biggest challenges facing caregivers and families is balancing the promotion of independence with the provision of protection.

Maintaining skills

Doing tasks

As the dementia progresses, people become slower and more disorganised in their approach to tasks. They cannot automatically recall what has to be done and even apparently simple tasks are extraordinarily difficult for them. It seems so much easier to allow others to take over and complete the task, but this deprives dementia sufferers of the satisfaction of getting things done and reinforces any feelings of uselessness and worthlessness. Patience is essential! People with dementia pick up on other people's frustration and become anxious themselves. Being anxious makes it even harder to carry out the task.

It may also be necessary for carers, family and friends to accept that the person has done a less-than-perfect job. If it is good enough, accept it. If you really need to patch things up, be tactful and subtle about it. Confronting people with dementia with their inadequacies will not help, especially if they cannot retain information long enough to learn from it.

If help is needed, it is better to offer to do things *with* people with dementia rather than *for* them. This keeps them involved and generates feelings of companionship, as demonstrated in the following example:

> *George and Edna have started to share the meal preparation. Edna has had trouble deciding what to have for dinner and in timing the cooking so that everything is ready to serve together. Between them, they work out what to eat. George picks out and measures the ingredients while Edna does the more straightforward things, such as peeling the potatoes, cutting the beans and mixing. They enjoy sharing the tasks. George is venturing into a new arena and Edna is pleased that she can continue to contribute usefully, but without having total responsibility for the outcome.*

Gentle reminders help overcome short-term memory loss. Break down complex chores, like cooking a meal, into simple parts. Make sure you give only one direction at a time, otherwise the person with dementia may get muddled. If understanding of language has diminished, it may be easier to gesture or demonstrate an action then just say it. It is important to focus on what the person can do, rather than what they cannot, and give encouragement and thanks when they are due.

Sometimes family members get annoyed and think that the person is just being lazy, but it is unlikely that someone who has always worked hard will suddenly become lazy in late life. Being unable to do what was once so easy is as upsetting for the person as it is for the relatives. Eroding someone's confidence by criticising or making demands of them will only make the situation worse.

Social skills

It is important for people with dementia and their carers to continue to socialise, otherwise isolation and loneliness set in. Apathy and withdrawal are common in moderate dementia. Going out to do the shopping, having a haircut or attending church or clubs keeps people involved in the local community.

Friends could take the person out to old haunts, which they otherwise couldn't get to or might lack the confidence to visit. A walk around the garden centre, a trip to a café for a cup of coffee, or a visit to the bowling green to watch a game, if playing has become too difficult, are all ideal outings for people with moderate Alzheimer's.

It is hard for people with dementia to cope with crowds, lots of noise and multiple conversations. Rowdy, multi-generational family gatherings, for all the pleasure they might bring, can be overwhelming. Too much stimulation can be distressing, though it is equally important that people with dementia are not left out. Ensure that a responsible relative keeps an eye on the person to ensure they are neither left alone nor exhausted by trying to keep up.

It might be necessary to explain to some key people in the community that a person with dementia has difficulties. For example, if the manager of the local restaurant is told of the person's trouble with crowds, he or she can suggest quiet times to come in or arrange seating at a table away from the busy areas.

Taking over

Dementia is a progressive condition and, despite every effort to maintain their skills, sooner or later the person will be unable to cope in some areas. This will happen very gradually. Ideally the main support person will be aware of the person's strengths and weaknesses, and will take over a task only when it is clearly beyond the person's capacity, or if they are asked for help.

Sometimes people struggle on, trying to do what they clearly cannot and becoming distressed by it. It is important to encourage such individuals to focus their attention on things they can accomplish. At the same time, the carer needs to take over what the person with dementia cannot do and this can require some delicate manoeuvring. Sometimes people are just anxious not to overburden a carer. In other cases, personal pride pushes them to continue doing something they have always done. It is so difficult to give up something you've always enjoyed doing well!

It is not always clear when a carer should take over a task, whether it even needs to be done or who should do it. How often should an older lady change her clothes or have a shower? Does it matter when she eats her main meal or how clean the house is? The best way to judge these issues might be to look at the standards prior to the onset of dementia. But what if people seem unaware that they are not maintaining previously kept standards? What if they deny the evidence of old food in the fridge and say they don't need help with the cleaning or shopping? It may be that the person with dementia is genuinely not aware that there are problems, or it might be that they are desperately trying to shore up their fading independence by refusing to acknowledge any need for help.

A flexible approach is best. Someone who refuses help at one time might accept it at another time, or from another person. Sometimes a suggestion needs to be phrased differently to be acceptable. For example, older people will often agree to a shower before visiting the doctor or going on a special outing. Clean clothes can be left out for after the bath or shower, and the dirty ones whisked out of sight for washing. Carers get very skilled at helping attend to the person's needs. Working with people with dementia certainly helps to clarify priorities and makes caregivers realise that much of what we are used to doing is not totally necessary. Examples of families adjusting their expectations of an Alzheimer's sufferer follow:

> *Mrs J. had always been very fussy about her appearance and her house, and had passed these values on to her children. Now living alone and suffering from moderate Alzheimer's, she is supported by her two daughters. They visit often, but their mother always says she is managing fine and does not want to put them out. Nevertheless, they usually bring some shopping when they come. While putting it away and making a cup of tea, they check for and dispose of any out-of-date food. They often give the bathroom a bit of a clean while they are in there. They have found that an upfront approach works if they see stains on their mother's clothes — they tell her about them and offer to take things home to wash. They have been discussing with her the idea of getting some help with showering, knowing she would find this less embarrassing coming from a professional caregiver than her family. After some soul-searching they have decided not to worry too much about the dust, as their mother seems unaware of it.*

Mr P. had always managed the finances and Mrs P. was reluctant to take them over, despite the fact that things were in a bit of a muddle. She had found unpaid bills and they had received a number of reminder notices. When she hesitantly approached her husband about this, he was angry that she questioned his abilities. She discussed the situation with her son and he arranged to spend time with his father once a month, going through the financial affairs. Mr P. agreed to this as a way of ensuring Mrs P. was looked after in future, should he be unable to do so. Father and son enjoyed their regular contact, and eventually Mr P. felt able to hand over the entire operation to his son.

It is difficult for children to reverse roles; that is, to begin parenting their parent. Likewise, if a husband (or wife) with dementia has been very domineering, it is hard for their spouse to begin to assert themselves late in life. The primary carer in these situations will need the backing of other family members, both emotionally and practically.

In more dire situations, such as when a person is driving dangerously or persistently setting fire to things on the stove, more coercive action may be required. Getting a professional, such as a doctor, social worker or community constable, to talk to the person with dementia sometimes helps. If the whole family is united in voicing their concerns and offering alternatives, the person might finally be convinced they need assistance.

What it is like for the person with dementia

At this stage it is often very difficult for a person with dementia to describe what is going on, but observers can sometimes see by their behaviour that, for such a person, the world is an unsafe, unfamiliar place. It is hard for them to know what to do in it. However, the person is still sensitive to the emotional tone of the environment and can be reassured by the presence of someone familiar, or frightened by an abrupt approach. Being hurried alarms such people because, although they may have received an explanation for the haste, they have forgotten it.

People with dementia may recognise clothes as things to be put on, but have forgotten the actions necessary for this. Or the clothes could look familiar, but they cannot remember what they are for. Life becomes puzzling and can be frightening if the person believes that some sort of trouble will result from failure to carry out instructions. It is a relief to have a gentle person give support.

What it is like for the family

By the time dementia has reached the moderate stage most families have come to accept that their relative has a progressive disease. They are usually brave, practical and resourceful, and deal with problems with grace and a sense of humour. There will be times when they are frightened or frustrated by some of the things their family member says or does. There will probably be disagreements as to the best way to handle things.

Sometimes people feel that they are losing the person they love, because although the person with dementia remains superficially polite and appropriate, the depth of spoken communication is lost. Different methods of communication need to be used to overcome this (see page 81).

There are many practical problems that have to be dealt with. As the moderate stage progresses, the person with dementia will need more and more help in day-to-day activities, such as cooking, choosing the right clothes and getting dressed, showering or shaving and dealing with bladder or bowel accidents. Some family members manage this well, but others find it too embarrassing. There is often an expectation that one person — the oldest daughter or the person with nursing training — will take over personal care. If this person is reluctantly pressed into the role as primary caregiver they are likely to become resentful and burned out. Additional sources of help, including from professional carers, should be sought before this stage is reached.

Cognitive changes

Memory loss

Memory loss becomes more marked in the moderate stage of dementia. It begins to extend further back, so that more than just short-term memory is affected. People with dementia might seem to be living in the past, and talk about their parents as if they are still alive or mistake their children for brothers or sisters.

Speech

Speech can either become very repetitive or the person can eventually stop saying much at all. The conversation below, taken from Margaret Forster's book *Have the Men had Enough?*[1] clearly shows this repetition, as Grandma talks to her granddaughter:

> *Grandma: Do you like school?*
>
> *Hannah: No.*
>
> *Grandma: I loved school.*
>
> *Hannah: Why did you leave at thirteen then?*

Grandma: Everyone did.

Hannah: No they didn't. Your sister stayed on.

Grandma: I loved school.

Hannah: So you say.

Grandma: Do you like school?

As the illness progresses, it becomes very difficult to string a sentence together. People may be left with only a few words, which have to suffice for a whole range of meanings.

Agnosia

Agnosia is the failure to recognise objects and to know what they are used for. People may puzzle over a toothbrush and try to use it as a comb. Familiar faces become unfamiliar and people with dementia may no longer recognise their home as such. This can be terrifying. They may not be able to be comforted by a lifelong spouse, or they might want to leave and go home even though they are already there.

Apraxia

Apraxia is the inability to carry out physical tasks despite having no physical problem that would prevent them from doing so. This is one of the things that makes dressing difficult. It becomes hard to know how to do such routine things as putting arms in sleeves or pulling on trousers. People may forget what order to put clothes on so, for example, they put a singlet on over their shirt. At this time the person needs supervision and perhaps practical help.

> Dressing most days is a reasonably happy and comic business. I am still far from sure which way round her underpants are supposed to go: we usually decide between us that it doesn't matter.
>
> IRIS, JOHN BAYLEY [2]

Emotional and psychological changes

The psychological effects of Alzheimer's disease are caused both by direct effects of brain damage and the sufferer's reaction to those changes. These changes occur in the context of the person's particular personality and are modified by that personality. For example, a person who has always tended to blame others will be more prone to suspiciousness, a shy person will increasingly withdraw from society. Changes include:

Anger and aggression: People are often angry because they are frightened or unable to understand what others want. Or they may be frustrated at their inability to explain what they want.

Apathy: The loss of motivation and drive suggests that the frontal lobe of the brain is affected. People withdraw when the demands of coping socially become too much. They can lose interest in sex and other activities.

Disinhibition: People with dementia may do things that are not socially acceptable, such as behaving in a sexually provocative manner or laughing at a funeral. They may strike out when frustrated.

Paranoid beliefs or suspiciousness: People who do not understand what is happening may try to explain their experiences by accusing others of being involved in some way. (A man who wet his bed explained this by saying aliens had interfered with him during the night.)

Misperceptions: People may see or hear one thing, but conclude that it is something else. Sometimes the family photos take on a life of their own, and a person feels there are crowds in the room or that meals must be prepared for these 'visitors'. A man may fail to recognise his own face in the mirror and become enraged, thinking that his wife has another man in the house.

Hallucinations: They may perceive something that is not there. For example, a woman may see her sister sitting in a chair and find this comforting. Another might complain that her stuffed animals move and poke their tongues out at her. Hallucinations can be of sound, smell, taste or touch. These experiences can lead to changes in behaviour; a woman may bang on the walls of the flat when she 'hears' the neighbours playing loud music; a man might smell leaking gas and repeatedly complain, though the gas company cannot detect anything wrong; a woman might refuse food that tastes odd because she thinks it is poisoned.

Depression is less prominent: The frequency of depression seems to diminish as people with dementia become less aware that there is something wrong and thus do not notice what they have lost.

Anxiety is expressed in different ways: People still get anxious but this anxiety is expressed in different ways, such as changed behaviour, as the ability to communicate verbally declines.

Changes in function and behaviour

People in the middle stage of Alzheimer's disease need help to manage daily chores. They may need reminders to eat, wash, dress and use the toilet. They may put themselves at risk because of forgetfulness; for example, by wandering outside inadequately clothed, leaving the stove on or letting predatory people into the house. They begin to lose basic hygiene skills at this time. Barry Reisberg's Functional Assessment Staging scale (below) sums up the changes in function at this stage.

MODERATE DEMENTIA

5. *Requires assistance in choosing proper clothing to wear for the day or season, e.g. patient may wear the same clothing repeatedly unless supervised.*
6. *(a) Requires actual physical help putting on clothes.*
   (b) Requires assistance to bathe properly.
   (c) Requires assistance to handle the mechanics of toileting (e.g. forgets to flush the toilet).
   (d) Urinary incontinence (occasionally or more frequently over past weeks).
   (e) Faecal incontinence (occasionally or more frequently over past weeks).

Functional Assessment Staging (FAST)

As their verbal communication skills deteriorate, people express their needs in other ways; for example, their insecurity may mean that they hate to let their spouse out of their sight, so follow him or her round closely. If they do not want to do something, they may physically resist or strike out at the person trying to get them to do it. These behaviours can be difficult for carers to understand and manage.

Other dementias

Vascular dementia

The progression of vascular dementia is unpredictable and may occur in abrupt steps. The cognitive changes depend on which part of the brain is damaged. As more brain tissue is lost and the changes become more widespread, vascular dementia begins to look more like Alzheimer's disease. One key difference is that people with vascular dementia often retain their insight through to this moderate stage, and are aware of their limitations. They may develop physical problems such as weakness or difficulty in walking if they have further additional strokes. They may also have seizures.

Lewy body dementia

People with Lewy body dementia also show an overall deterioration. There are fluctuations in performance, but the good periods are not so lucid and may be less frequent. Short-term memory, which was initially preserved, begins to fail. Visual hallucinations, falls and difficulty judging distance remain a problem as do the Parkinsonian symptoms of stiffness, tremor, slowness and difficulty in walking.

Frontal lobe dementia

As frontal lobe dementias progress they too begin to look like Alzheimer's as more of the brain becomes involved. Because younger people get this disorder it tends to progress more quickly.

Things to do

- Learn to communicate with the person with dementia in ways other than through speech. Let all carers (both formal and informal) know the sort of signs the person uses and how to interpret them.
- Enjoy together what you can; laugh at the funny things that happen.
- Assess what extra support might be needed, now and in the future; such as help with bathing and dressing, day or respite care, incontinence pads, etc.
- Take over tasks as necessary, but try to share them around so that no one is overburdened.
- Find out what help is available, through Alzheimer's New Zealand, the public health system, privately and from family and friends.
- Get help sooner rather than later so that the person with dementia gets used to other people coming in and the carer avoids getting exhausted.
- Accept that other carers might not be as good as you and might need some training, but that they will probably be good enough. The person

with dementia will get used to them and may even begin to enjoy the change of company.

- Make contingency plans should the main caregiver suddenly be unable to continue.
- Talk to the bank manager if the person is having trouble with money, or the police if there is a tendency for them to wander.
- If you are the main carer, make sure you take time for yourself.
- Find a sympathetic support person with whom you can share your frustrations, anger or sadness, or just have a break from responsibilities.

Where to seek support and advice

Family and friends are likely to be your main source of support. Alzheimer's New Zealand can provide group support through their regional branches and information through their website, leaflets or phone service. Your general practitioner should be able to put you in contact with Needs Assessment and Service Coordination (NASC) services to arrange for help at home.

If you are already involved with the local older people's services in the public health system, you can contact your case worker through the hospital.

A psychiatrist with experience and interest in dementia can be contacted via the GP if the person has delusions or hallucinations, or is behaving in a way that is difficult for carers to cope with.

Remember, it is really important for caregivers to look after themselves. The person with dementia depends on the carer. Bravely struggling on without assistance is not admirable, it is foolish. The person with dementia will sense when the person they love is stressed, exhausted or irritable, and become distressed in turn. Then the quality of life for both people deteriorates.

In summary

In middle-stage dementia, patients begin to need more help and the caregiver requires more support. Family and friends need to be involved and professional care services might be used. The next chapter looks at advanced dementia.

References

[1] Forster, Margaret, *Have the Men Had Enough?* Chatto & Windus, London, 1989, p. 22.

[2] Bayley, John, *Iris: A Memoir of Iris Murdoch,* Duckworth Publications, London, 1998, p. 81.

Chapter 6

Severe dementia

But now I'm an old woman,
So I want the last word;
There is no such thing as time —
Only this very minute
And I'm in it.
Thank the Lord.

JOYCE GRENFELL [1]

A person with severe dementia has become dependent on others for day-to-day care. This is roughly 8–10 years after the onset of Alzheimer's disease, though it can be earlier in faster forms of dementia (in younger people) or later if the progression is slower, such as in vascular dementia.

Alzheimer's disease

At this point, the person is very disabled. Speech is badly affected, other skills are lost and the person has become more frail; the disease wastes the body as well as the brain. People close to the patient sometimes feel that the person they loved is no longer there or is just a shell. Others, however, feel that they can communicate at some level and still detect the essence of the person they love. Some people continue to care for the person on the basis of memories of what he or she was like. It may not be so difficult for the person with dementia:

> Despite her illness, or maybe somehow because of it, Margo is one of the happiest people I have known. There is something graceful about the degeneration her mind is undergoing, leaving her carefree, always cheerful. Do her problems, whatever she may perceive them to be, simply fail to make it to the worry centers of her brain?
>
> A PIECE OF MY MIND [2]

While it can be deeply satisfying and meaningful to care for a loved person who is now very dependent, it is also physically and emotionally tiring. Many caregivers are old themselves, and do not have the physical strength to nurse someone who is losing their mobility. Sleepless nights take their toll, and the 24-hour demands of care restrict and isolate the carer. Most people with severe Alzheimer's disease will be approaching, or already in, residential or hospital care.

Communication

When the disease has robbed someone of most or all of their words, and understanding is limited, carers need to be creative and use all the other forms of communication at their disposal. Interaction with a person with dementia can occur in many different forms. These include:

Tone and volume of voice: People with dementia can tell the difference between a gentle reassuring tone and a harsh or bossy voice, and react accordingly.

Gesture: The carer's gestures, along with words, help relay a message to the person with dementia. The carer should also learn to interpret the gestures made by the person with dementia.

Posture: Caregivers may be able to read the mood of a person with dementia from their posture, for example, upright and alert or angry, or slumped, cowed or frightened. Conversely, the stance of the caregiver can convey the caregiver's mood — positive, negative, aggressive or relaxed.

Position: Invasion of someone's personal space can be threatening, yet keeping at a distance can seem cold or rejecting. Different cultures and individuals tolerate different degrees of physical closeness and the carer needs to be aware of personal preferences.

Movement: Sudden movements by carers can be frightening so should be avoided. The person with dementia may be trying to communicate something by pacing or making repetitive movements.

Facial expression: A person with dementia will show pain, fear, anger or pleasure by their facial expression, and may also be able to read these signs on a carer's face.

Touch: Touch can be gentle or rough, urgent or reassuring. A person with dementia may use touch to indicate their needs, for example, pulling on an arm to show the caregiver something.

Shared sensual pleasures: Enjoying music, a spa bath or a walk outside are all ways of communicating companionship and warmth.

Understanding the person over a long period of time: As a carer spends more time with the person they will grow to understand their needs, habits and desires; for example, they may know that a person who is agitated after lunch is tired and needs a rest.

Nevertheless, speech is used as the main mode of communication for as long as possible. There are many suggestions for improving verbal communication with people with dementia as they lose the ability to comprehend others and to express themselves. One of these is the FOCUSED method.[3]

F= Face to face

1. *Face the person directly*
2. *Attract the person's attention*
3. *Maintain eye contact*

O= Orientation

1. *Orient the person by repeating key words several times*
2. *Repeat sentences exactly*
3. *Give the person time to comprehend what you have to say*

C= Continuity

1. *Continue the same topic of conversation for as long as possible*
2. *Prepare the person if a new topic must be introduced*

U= Unsticking

1. *Help the person to become 'unstuck' when he or she uses a word incorrectly, by suggesting the correct or missing word*
2. *Repeat the person's sentence using the correct or missing word*
3. *Ask, 'Do you mean . . .?'*

S= Structure

1. *Structure your questions to give the person a choice of response*
2. *Provide only two or three options at a time*
3. *Provide options that the person would like*

E= Exchange

1. *Keep up the normal exchange of ideas we find in conversation*
2. *Begin conversations with pleasant topics*
3. *Ask easy questions that the person can answer*
4. *Give the person clues as to how to answer*

D= Direct

1. *Keep sentences short, simple and direct (subject, verb, object)*
2. *Use and repeat nouns rather than pronouns (for example, say, 'could you give me the plate, please', rather than 'please give it to me')*
3. *Use hand signals, pictures and facial expressions.*

What it is like for the person

Obviously it is very hard for us to understand what it is like to have severe dementia. Even with careful attempts to understand communication, we often get it wrong when trying to work out what the person is experiencing. He or she does not recover to tell us what it was like. Any reports are, at best, informed guesses, attempts to read meaning from behaviour, physical and facial expressions and the occasional word. The person with dementia often seems to be unaware that there is anything wrong and this, presumably, reduces their sense of loss. In the following example, a daughter reflects on what life is like for her parents, both of whom have dementia:

> *They must feel so foolish, so inadequate. That's what frightens people. Yes, you try to put yourself in their position, but sometimes you can't believe it, every day's the same. And then you realise the horrible part is that you can't take them out, they can't go for a walk, so then they are housebound, and then they can't walk in the house, they can't eat, just have no idea how to get it (the fork) up there . . .*

The person with dementia may exist in a world of sights, sounds, smells and touch; sensations that perhaps mean very little in the intellectual sense, but are still emotionally important and able to promote comfort or discomfort. A soft blanket, a warm hug, a gentle breeze or some pleasant music must be better than the pressure of a hard chair, loud noises, unpleasant smells or being handled roughly. Although their communication skills deteriorate, people with severe dementia still appear to enjoy familiar songs, poems and prayers. Surprisingly, even people who haven't spoken for a long time will suddenly join in the chorus of an old song or hymn.

What it is like for the family

It is hard for the family to know how much to read into their relative's non-verbal signs and how much they interpret correctly. It is very difficult to watch someone deteriorate to the point that they forget their spouse's name or confuse him or her with their own parents. Perhaps that isn't too bad; at least the person sees the spouse as someone who is loving and caring.

It can be upsetting if the person seems to be suffering in some way; for example, if they are calling out or agitated. It may be difficult to find the cause of their distress. If the person is in residential care, it can be frustrating for staff trying to interpret the person's needs. The family, however, know the patient best and are most likely to know what the person with dementia is trying to communicate.

Tom Kitwood, a psychologist and dementia researcher, believes that the family is able to see through to the essential person despite the severe dementia.

> Is it possible then, that family caregivers are more attentive than others to the fragile clues of selfhood? Is it possible that in their attentive, caring presence, caregivers really do see some core of a self that less present observers would dismiss as fantasy, denial or attribution? [4]

Caring for someone who is gradually losing their skills is very sad. However, some people are able to make some meaning out of this, perhaps feeling that the ultimate gift they can give is to care for the one they love most in the world. A family can often pull together and support each other, and this generates a closeness that might not otherwise have developed.

Cognitive changes

In severe dementia the person is deeply forgetful and may not be able to follow any instructions at all because the information is lost from memory almost as soon as it is received. People with severe dementia cannot keep up with the time of day nor the date and may be unaware of where they are (especially if they have recently been moved to a new situation). They will gradually lose the ability to name and recognise even those people who are nearest and dearest, though there may still be some awareness that people are familiar.

Long-term memory is more affected as the dementia progresses. Time seems to roll back. The elderly woman who, at an earlier stage, worried about cooking for the family when they got home from school, might now believe her own mother is looking after her. For most, childhood memories are happy and peaceful, but those who had a difficult childhood may become anxious. Eventually, even these memories seem to pass.

Emotional and psychological changes

Emotions *seem* to become less complicated in those with severe dementia, who appear to experience only contentment or non-specific distress. They may show minimal reactions to their surroundings, although still draw back from pain, or relax when soothed. The agitation and depression of earlier stages may mercifully lessen. The hallucinations and delusions present in the moderate stage may be less obvious, and medication used to control these can be reduced or stopped. Some people seem to retain certain elements of their personality right until the end, as a daughter describes in the following example:

> *I think in the back of his mind (and I know you'll probably think I'm nuts), but I know in the back of his mind, even though he was impaired, that his first thought was always his wife. Is she all right? And even towards the end, a couple of weeks before he died, he would say something to me about Mum.*

Changes in function and behaviour

By definition, severe dementia is the stage when the affected people are no longer able to care for themselves. They eventually lose their ability to speak and may wander aimlessly, though eventually they also lose their ability to walk. The normal sleep pattern goes and people may sleep more during the day. Incontinence becomes a problem. At the terminal stages of dementia, there is often weight loss. This is part of the illness and not just related to difficulties with eating.

SEVERE DEMENTIA

6. *(d) Urinary incontinence (occasionally or more frequently over past weeks).*
   (e) Faecal incontinence (occasionally or more frequently over past weeks).

7. *(a) Speech limited to about six words in the course of an average day.*
(b) Speech limited to the use of a single intelligible word in an average day.
(c) Ambulatory ability lost (cannot walk without personal assistance).
(d) Cannot sit up without assistance.
(e) Loss of ability to smile.
(f) Loss of ability to hold up head independently.

Functional Assessment Staging (FAST)

Other dementias

Vascular dementia

It can take up to 20 years before the end-stage of vascular dementia is reached. This, however, depends on the rate and amount of brain damage, so this stage might be reached a lot sooner.

Because the damage in vascular dementia is patchy, there may be 'islands' of functioning still left, even as the vascular dementia reaches the late stage. For example, the person may be able to comprehend more than others expect, although their speech may be limited.

Lewy body dementia

Lewy body dementia tends to progress faster than Alzheimer's disease. The condition becomes severe after 5–8 years. As the severity increases, the illness becomes more difficult to distinguish from Alzheimer's and the hallucinations and fluctuations in performance become less marked.

Frontotemporal dementia

As brain damage becomes more widespread the frontotemporal dementias become difficult to distinguish from other dementias. Because the progress is usually faster than Alzheimer's disease, the final stage is reached sooner.

Physical changes in severe dementia

In the final stages of dementia, the physical care of the person becomes the prime consideration.

Bladder and bowel problems

Most people in the end stages of dementia lose bladder control, and frequently bowel control as well. Initially, people are embarrassed by incontinence and may try to hide evidence of the problem or clean up themselves, but later they are less aware of what has happened. Reminding people to go to the toilet or taking them there regularly can prevent accidents and maintain their pride. A large sign on the toilet door can help them find their way to the toilet. People with dementia can still associate the sight of the toilet with passing water and thus use it appropriately. Sometimes astute caregivers realise that certain signs, such as restlessness, indicate a desire to urinate.

If people are left sitting around in wet clothing they can develop skin problems, hence the need to keep them dry. There are now some excellent incontinence products, which can be used at night or when going out. (Sometimes people find these pants bulky and annoying and take them off to indicate this.) Catheters are rarely used, except when there are additional problems, such as urine retention caused by an enlarged prostate. Many District Health Boards (and some other services) employ a continence nurse who has expertise in managing these problems and can recommend suitable incontinence products. General practitioners or hospital-based services can put caregivers in contact with the continence service.

Constipation can cause discomfort and increased confusion, so carers need to be alert to this problem. Apparent diarrhoea, with runny stools which leak out, can be caused by a blockage further up the bowel (this is known as 'constipation with overflow'). It is important to check that this is not the problem before giving anti-diarrhoea medication, which would make the situation worse. General practitioners, a practice nurse or a district nurse can help with treatment of constipation, though most carers can work out a suitable regime using stool softeners such as kiwifruit or Lactulose.

Hygiene

People with advanced dementia need assistance with personal hygiene. If the person stands in the shower (or sits in the bath), but does not wash, the caregiver will have to instruct them what to do, give them a soapy flannel or actually wash them. This invasion of privacy can be difficult for both the family and the person with dementia. Sometimes it is more comfortable for everyone if a paid caregiver comes in a few times a week to give the person a shower. If the person is not particularly active and not incontinent, a shower a couple of times a week is probably sufficient. Having a bath or shower can be a scary business if the patient has forgotten what it is all about. Going into a small space like a shower can be confusing if the person cannot judge distance and depth. Keeping a plastic chair in the shower can make showering easier if the person is unsteady. Carefully explaining each step and guiding the person in a calm manner makes this task easier.

Loss of mobility and falling

Falls become more common in the later stages of dementia. People bump into things or lose their balance and fall over, but they are unaware of the risk so keep on walking around. Restricting the person's movements to keep them safe often makes them agitated. The family usually has to accept that there is a risk of falls and should keep a close watch on the patient to reduce the frequency of these. A person with severe dementia is unlikely to learn how to use a walking stick or frame if they are not already used to them. Hip protectors, which are worn in specially designed underpants, help to prevent fractures should the person fall (they can be sourced through www.impactwear.co.nz). However, some people find these strange and uncomfortable and object to wearing them. Reduce the risk of falls by making sure there are no rugs or stray cords to trip over. Install stair-rails and grab-rails by the bath and toilet. Check with the doctor that prescribed medication will not cause unsteadiness (most tranquillising drugs cause drowsiness and affect balance).

It can be difficult to get people up off the ground once they have fallen. A physiotherapist can advise the best methods. Often, more than one person is needed to lift someone who has fallen. If you can't lift them immediately, keep the person warm by covering them with a blanket and putting a pillow under their head before seeking help from neighbours, family or anyone available. (I know of one person who called in the strong-looking men who were mending her road.) It is okay to call for an ambulance if someone falls. The ambulance crew will pick the person up and check them over for injury.

Some people with dementia retain the ability to walk for a long time, losing it only when they fall ill with another injury or disease. In these cases, the family can continue to help the person to move around, but to avoid the risk of injuring themselves or the person with dementia it is wise to get advice from a nurse or physiotherapist. When necessary, a physiotherapist can advise on the use of a wheelchair (which may be lent out by the hospital or hired from private sources). Often at this stage of the illness the person with dementia will have lost weight, which makes it easier to transfer them in and out of chairs. If the person is heavy, two people will be needed to move them safely.

Even when a person cannot move around freely, at least some of their day can be spent sitting in the company of others. If the person spends most of the day sitting or lying down, seek professional advice on gentle exercises to keep their limbs flexible. If their joints remain flexible it is easier for patients to be washed and moved around.

Skin care

Once the ability to walk or move around has been lost, people need careful nursing to avoid developing pressure sores. People normally make dozens of little movements in order to keep comfortable when they are sitting or lying down. For people with dementia, messages about discomfort do not get through to the brain and the person can remain motionless for long periods. This puts pressure on one spot (usually the buttocks, heels, or shoulder blades), which can cause the skin to break down. If the person is being cared for at home, visiting district nurses can help to prevent or treat pressure sores and also teach the family how to do this. There are now excellent air- or fluid-filled pads and mattresses available which can be placed in chairs or on beds. These distribute the person's weight more evenly, reducing pressure on the areas that bear weight when someone is sitting or lying down for a long time. Sheepskin slippers and elbow pads protect heels and elbows.

As people age their skin gets thinner and tears more easily, even with slight stress. People also bruise more easily, so they need to be handled very gently. This can be difficult, at times, particularly if they are resisting care.

Eating and drinking

People with dementia gradually lose their table manners and then their ability to use cutlery. If they are too restless to stay at the table long enough to eat, provide frequent finger food rather than worrying about the niceties of sitting down to a full meal. People who are moving all the time need sufficient calories to maintain their weight. Easily digested, high-calorie drinks such as Complan, Ensure, Sustagen, Fortisip and Thrive can be bought at a pharmacy or obtained free (apart from dispensing charges), after some form-filling, from a specialist doctor. These are expensive items, so talk to a dietician or GP before committing to paying for them long term. Carers come up with their own ingenious ideas for getting food and fluids into their family members.

We couldn't get her to drink at that time and all of a sudden it clicked. We gave Mum a cup and saucer and it came back to her like that. I got out an old, beautiful bone china set. And I got out these little glasses that were crystal. Fine crystal, not cut, fine rim. She drank everything out of those.

People in the very late stages of dementia may no longer recognise food as something that is meant to be eaten. They may not realise that they are hungry and resist the carer who is trying to feed them, by turning away or pushing the plate off the table. Sometimes, even if the food does get into their mouth, they forget how to chew or swallow and spit it out or let it dribble away. Feeding someone with end-stage dementia can be a very time-consuming, messy and frustrating business. People almost always lose weight in the end stages of Alzheimer's disease. This is not just a result of their difficulties in eating and feeding, but part of the illness itself.

Dental care

Dental hygiene is important, but it is sometimes very difficult to clean the teeth of people with dementia. They can develop gum inflammation or abscesses, and the infection can spread beyond their mouth. In earlier stages of the illness people may still be able to clean their teeth if reminded and assisted. Later the caregiver will have to do it. One approach is for the patient to sit in a dining chair with the carer behind them. The carer supports the patient against their body, cradles their head in one arm, and uses the other hand to brush their teeth. Some find an electric toothbrush works well. Antiseptic wafers that dissolve on the person's tongue or mouthwash obtainable from the chemist or dentist also do a reasonable job. Or you may find other ways, as shown in the example below:

They just did the front bit and would say, 'Right J., you can swish your mouth out,' and we would make these noises, because she could hear that, but she couldn't really understand. They would get the toothbrush and do each side and in the end, she would be waiting so that she could just swish the water.

A change in behaviour, such as refusal to eat or to wear dentures or pulling at the face or mouth, might indicate the patient has dental problems.

In some areas there are dentists who are experts in dealing with people with dementia. The dental department at your regional hospital should know who is available. Some private and public hospital dentists will visit people in their own home or residential care facilities (at a cost if the person does not qualify for a subsidy).

Other problems

If people spend a lot of time lying down, they are more likely to get pneumonia because they cannot properly clear secretions from their lungs. Once swallowing becomes difficult, there is a risk of inhaling food and getting a chest infection as a result.

It is hard to tell if a person with severe dementia is in pain. If they have any condition, such as arthritis, that might be causing pain or discomfort, it is best to give suitable pain relief anyway. However, various pain scales, such as the Abbey Pain Scale, have been developed to measure pain in people who cannot communicate verbally.

Seizures (fits) occasionally occur at this stage. You won't be able to stop a seizure; the main goal is to prevent the person being injured (and not get too alarmed yourself). If you can, once the shaking has stopped, lie the person on their side in the recovery position. One seizure is not usually life-threatening, but the person should be checked by their GP, who will decide whether it is worth treating them with anticonvulsant medication.

In the terminal stages of dementia normal sleep patterns are lost and people often sleep a lot.

Things to do

Carers at home will need a lot of support when the patient develops severe dementia. Although the family may be able to manage just using its own resources, there are plenty of community services available to help with ongoing care. As many of these services are free, it seems a good idea to take advantage of them. Your GP or specialist old-age service can arrange for an assessment and for assistance to be put in place. There is sometimes a delay, so ask for help as soon as you think you might need it.

If someone is in residential care, the family still has an important role to play. Sometimes people feel excluded once they hand over their loved one to the care of professionals. It is part of the professional's role to involve family members and not to intimidate them. Chapter 13 looks at how families and care organisations can (and must) work together in the best interests of the people with dementia.

Where to seek support and advice

Alzheimer's New Zealand groups can offer support to families and carers at this difficult stage. They can also provide information on handling various issues. Your GP or old-age service should be able to assist you by referring the patient to the Needs Assessment Services for different forms of practical support.

In summary

This can be a difficult time, as the person deteriorates physically and needs more and more help. Communication can be a challenge. However, the person with dementia may be happy enough and many people find meaning and deep satisfaction in providing care for someone with severe dementia.

References

[1] Grenfell, Joyce, 'Time', from *Stately as a Galleon*, Chivers Press, Bath, 1978.

[2] Firlik, Andrew D., 'A piece of my mind: Margo's logo', *Journal of the American Medical Association*, 265 (2): 201, 1991.

[3] Ripich, D. & Wykle, M., 'Developing health care professionals' communication skills with Alzheimer's disease patients.' Paper presented at the annual meeting of the American Society on Aging, San Francisco. Post, Stephen G., *The Moral Challenge of Alzheimer's Disease*, 1995, pp. 25–26. (Reprinted with permission of John Hopkins University Press, Baltimore.)

[4] Kitwood, Tom, *Dementia Reconsidered: The person comes first*, Open University Press, Buckingham, 1997.

Chapter 7

Therapies for dementia

Successful treatment of patients with dementia requires a broad range of tasks . . . these tasks help to maximise the patient's level of function and to ensure the safety and comfort of patients and their families in the context of living with a difficult disease.

AMERICAN PSYCHIATRIC ASSOCIATION [1]

There are many ways to improve the lives of people with dementia. Not every approach suits every person. What helps any individual will depend on that person's character and preferences, their living situation, the support available and the stage of the dementia. In this chapter, I will describe a variety of non-medical approaches, some accepted and well-proven, others of less certain usefulness. (Chapter 8 focuses on medication.) I have also listed the sorts of people who might be able to help. Trying a particular treatment should be viewed as an experiment. If it helps, that's great; if not, something has been learned. When trying to find a solution to a problem, the person with dementia must be respected and included in the decision-making process.

Tom Kitwood, working in the 1990s, introduced the concept of 'person-centred care'.[2] This moved the emphasis of management away from the illness (dementia) to the person who had it, and their surroundings. He tried to understand what effect the illness had on the *person* suffering it, that is, the person's experience of dementia. He felt that the main goal of care was to help people with dementia to stay being themselves — that is, to retain their 'personhood'.

Kitwood studied the way that other people interact with someone with dementia. Some interactions improve the person's wellbeing, others make it worse. To get a taste for his approach, here are three examples taken from his list of seventeen behaviours by other people which undermine the personhood of someone with dementia:

Disempowerment: not allowing a person to use the abilities that they do have; failing to help them complete actions that they have initiated. For example, a woman is very slow at peeling the potatoes, so her husband takes the peeler off her and finishes the job himself.

Ignoring: behaving (in conversation or action) in the presence of a person as if they were not there. An example is two nurses discussing their weekends over the top of a patient while they wash his back in bed.

Stigmatisation: the person with dementia becomes strange, alien, a diseased object, an outcast. Old friends call in once or twice after the diagnosis, but eventually the visits drop off completely because they feel uncomfortable and don't know what to say.

Tom Kitwood called this kind of behaviour 'malignant social psychology' and developed methods to allow carers to recognise and avoid such interactions. If these methods are used, not only are people with dementia more relaxed and happier, but they can even regain skills that have been lost, a process Dr Kitwood called rementing.

I cannot hope to explain his methods of person-centred care in a few paragraphs, but interested people could read his book *Dementia Reconsidered*. I hope the spirit of the person-centred approach imbues this book.

Psychological approaches

Memory aids

There are three stages of forming a memory: learning or registration, storage and recall (see chapter 1). We are not able to do much about the storage stage, but may well be able to improve learning and recall. In general, we know that stress or worry (including worrying about your memory) makes it harder to remember things. We need to concentrate on one thing at a time if we want to remember it, and avoid distractions. Having a routine and being well organised makes it easier to recall where things are or what you are meant to be doing. These comments (as well as most of the suggestions that follow) apply to everyone, not just to people who know they are forgetful.

Here are some general suggestions for improving memory.

Finding things (including finding your way)

Organisation and aids

- Have set places to keep things; for example, your glasses by the bed, the keys near the door.
- Write a list of the things you tend to lose and where you might have put them; for example, your glasses might be in the bathroom or on the

coffee table. Put the list in a prominent place.
- Label cupboards with a list of the things inside them.
- Label the things you might lose (like your umbrella) with your name and phone number, so that people can return them to you if you leave them behind.
- If you go out, put the things you brought with you in an obvious place; for example, leave your coat near the front door, keep your bag within view.
- Count the number of things you took out with you. Count them on departure to make sure you have them all. (I do this already, when I go to work; six things: wallet, keys, lunch, ID tag, phone and . . . something else?)
- When travelling, look at the map before you leave or get someone to write down the directions. Include landmarks such as schools, petrol stations, etc.
- As you travel, make a note of what you are passing so you can remember the way back.
- Write down the phone number of the person you are going to see. You can call them if you get lost.

Attention, learning, registration

These strategies help register information.
- Concentrate when you put something away.
- Give yourself a reason as to why you are putting it there. I put the scissors in the top drawer because I use them often and can get them out easily.
- Make a connection between the item and the place; for example, if you are parking your car on the fifth floor of the car park visualise your hand with five fingers on the steering wheel. Some car parks make it easy by naming the floors after places ('I left my car in Napier') or giving them colours ('my white car is in the red car park . . . cherry ice-cream').

Recalling

If you have forgotten where something is, there are ways to jog your memory.
- Go back in your mind to when you last remember having the item.
- Pretend you are putting the item away for the first time . . . where would you put it?
- Look at your list of usual hiding places for that item.
- Relax. Do you really need it now? Is there a substitute? Getting upset won't help your memory.

Remembering to do things

Organisation and aids

- Use a calendar, diary or electronic aid. Carry a notebook (or use your phone) to note down what you need to do as it occurs to you, and refer to it regularly. Write your instructions for the day on a whiteboard.
- Leave 'Post-it' notes around the house and on the door so that you see them as you go out.
- Connect the task with something that is already routine for you; for example, leave any pills you need to take by your toothbrush.
- Put a rubber band round your wrist, change your watch to your other arm, write a message on your palm.
- Put things in your way so you can't avoid seeing them; for example, leave the letters you need to post by the door.
- Set an alarm to go off at the time you are supposed to do something (or get someone else to remind you).

Attention, learning, registration

- Repeat what you have to do several times and picture yourself doing it.
- Associate what you have to do with something else; for example, if there are several things to do, think of a story that links them.
- Try to remember things in groups; for example, all the cleaning products you need, things to do for the family.
- Regularly think through the things that have to be done to reinforce them in your memory.

Recalling

- Where were you when you thought of doing what it was that you've now forgotten? Go back there if possible.
- Refer to your list. See if you have checked off everything that needed doing.
- Talk to yourself as you do things, for example, 'I've locked the door'. You may remember saying that sentence even if you forget that you locked the door.

Remembering what people tell you

Organisation and aids

- Write things down.
- Put it in your computer or cellphone.

Attention, learning, registration

- Repeat what you've heard said. If it is a name you want to remember, use it as often as you can in the conversation.
- Use initials to make words; for example, if you are asked to buy Cereal, Apples, Bread and Shampoo, you could make the word CABS and associate it with the taxi stand outside the supermarket.
- With names, you might want to associate the person with someone else you know; for example, 'Elizabeth' with the queen. This is especially useful if your Elizabeth has regal bearing.
- Numbers, particularly phone numbers, are difficult to remember. They often fall into groups that are easier to recall; for example, for the number 230 1843: 230 can be recalled as the time 2.30 (when you go to the dentist) and 1843 as 3 years after the Treaty of Waitangi was signed. (Sometimes it is more realistic to write it down if possible!)
- You may be able to associate something about a person's appearance with their name; for example, Pretty Priscilla . . . lives up to her name.

Recalling

- Think of the situation you were in when told something. Imagine you are there or go there again if possible.
- Try to associate the message or name with other things, or remember how you were feeling at the time.
- Don't panic. It is always okay to ask for the information again . . . 'Your name has slipped my mind . . .' 'What was it you asked me to do?' After all, busy or otherwise distracted people often don't remember things too well. It's not such a big deal to acknowledge you've forgotten something.
- Ask other people for their ideas.

Something many people find very helpful is being a member of a group where they can share practical hints on how to cope with poor memory.

> *One man who had dementia became very anxious when his wife was out, because he couldn't remember when she would be back. Another man told him how to overcome the problem. He had bought a cheap watch that could be set to count down the minutes until his wife's intended return. He only had to look at it to be reassured that she wasn't late and would be back within a certain time.*

Behaviour modification therapy

Behaviour modification therapy is a formal therapy, normally both planned and provided by a psychologist. Essentially, behaviour therapy looks at incidents or situations that trigger unwanted behaviour (such as aggression or calling out), defines exactly what the behaviour is and how people respond to it. Then a plan is developed to lessen the behaviour by stopping the triggers and making sure that the response does not encourage (reinforce) the unwanted behaviour. For example: a woman in a rest home calls out frequently because she is bored (trigger). Staff go to see what she wants, and she is no longer bored (reinforcement) and stops calling out. She starts calling out again when they leave. In this case, dealing with the trigger (boredom) is the humane thing to do. Not reinforcing the behaviour by responding to her calls might also mean that she eventually quietens down. However, she would then have to develop some other way of relieving her boredom (perhaps by hitting the man in the next chair).

If behaviour modification is not carried out carefully, the unwanted behaviour may be replaced with another, perhaps even more challenging, behaviour. Carers sometimes carry out their own informal behaviour modification; for example, by ignoring a particular behaviour or changing the circumstances to prevent it occurring.

Cognitive behavioural therapy

Cognitive behavioural therapy (CBT) is a form of psychological therapy used widely in New Zealand to treat anxiety and depression. It can be used to help people with mild dementia who are anxious or depressed, and carers can use CBT to help them cope better.

According to CBT, people's feelings are influenced by the way they think and by what they do. Their thoughts are based on their beliefs about themselves, the world and the future. Their actions may reinforce negative views of themselves. It is possible to change the way people feel by changing both their underlying beliefs and the actions they take as a result of these.

For example, a caregiver who has just shouted at her husband might think, 'I'm a terrible carer . . .'. The belief behind this is 'I should always be calm and understanding, no matter what . . .'. The resulting feelings are of guilt and despair. CBT asks the carer to examine her belief. How can anyone expect to always keep calm under such demanding circumstances? If the carer judges herself less harshly she will be less likely to suffer from the feelings of guilt and despair. She may also recognise that she needs to do some of the things she enjoys and feels fulfilled in doing; for example, taking more exercise, visiting friends, doing a hobby (this is the behavioural part of CBT).

A woman who is newly diagnosed with dementia might think, 'Oh no, I'm going to end up in a mental hospital like my grandmother . . .'. Her underlying belief is that the diagnosis means she will end up in demeaning and humiliating circumstances. The belief can be challenged by becoming informed about recent advances in dementia care and by making decisions about what can be done now to arrange for the sort of future she would choose.

Validation therapy

In validation therapy, the carer or other therapist acknowledges that the emotions of people with dementia are real to them and responds on a feeling level rather than trying to reason with them. The therapist tries to understand how the person sees things and what they are feeling. When people are accepted and their feelings acknowledged they feel more alive, connected and real, and more of a person.

> *Mrs B. gets agitated in the afternoon and paces around the rest home, looking for her mother. Instead of telling her that her mother died years ago, the staff talk to Mrs B. about her mother and how much she misses her. They recognise that Mrs B. is feeling lost and bewildered and wants someone to comfort and protect her.*
>
> *They give her a cuddle, reassure her that she is safe there and tell her that they are going to look after her. Only when she is feeling more secure do they try to get her involved in another activity.*

Some people seem to be instinctively good at validation therapy, but we can all benefit from training and learn by experience.

Reality orientation

The goal of reality orientation therapy is to increase the awareness of the person with dementia — if they are aware of their surroundings they can be more independent and in control. The patient is told about current happenings such as the day, month, year, place and weather. Various aids such as flashcards with pictures of common objects — or noticeboards with the day, date and weather posted on them — can be used to help keep language and recognition skills. Therapy can be done in group sessions or on a continuous basis by caregivers.

There is evidence that this approach improves thinking, memory and behaviour. Many care institutions use some aspects of reality orientation, often by having up-to-date information written on a prominent whiteboard. Decorations and celebrations of significant events, such as Easter, Valentine's Day or 'important' rugby matches, all help keep long-term residents in touch with what is happening.

Reality orientation is less popular than it once was. This form of therapy needs to be used carefully otherwise it can repeatedly confront people who have dementia with evidence of their memory loss. This can have a devastating effect on their self-esteem. If people's current circumstances are unpleasant, it may be an unkindness to keep them aware of this. However, it is worrying to visit homes or hospitals where there are no clocks or calendars and it is difficult to see what the weather is like. It is not surprising when people living in such places are disorientated. A degree of reality orientation is important, but the method needs to be used sensitively.

Reminiscence therapy

Reminiscence therapy involves short sessions using slides, photos or other objects from the past to stimulate conversation and memories. A trained worker encourages groups of people with dementia to talk about old times. As long-term memory is intact until late in the illness, most people can join in. This can be stimulating and enjoyable and reduces the withdrawal that occurs in many people with dementia. I recently overheard a group of women talking about their first ball gowns. This evoked wonderful memories of swirling skirts, rustling taffeta and orchid sprays.

An alternative approach is life-review therapy, which is a form of reminiscence, usually done by an individual under the guidance of a therapist. The goal is to put memories in some sort of context and come to terms with the life the person has had.

'Alternative' treatments

Acupuncture

Traditional Chinese acupuncture can be used to reduce pain, relax muscles and relieve stress. In New Zealand, acupuncture may be performed by physiotherapists, GPs or experts in Chinese medicine. Members of the New Zealand Register of Acupuncturists are listed in the Yellow Pages. As with all therapies, ask how long the session will take, what will happen and what the cost will be.

Aromatherapy

Aromatherapy involves the use of oils from plants to treat symptoms of dementia. The oil can be diffused in the air, added to a bath or rubbed on the skin as part of a massage (you may need to dilute it first). Many people with dementia lose their sense of smell, so it appears that something other than the perfume of the oil has a positive effect.

Lavender oil can have a calming effect and make people feel relaxed and content. It can be used during the day or at night, when a few drops on the bedsheets can help people sleep. Citrus oil is said to improve mood and provide extra energy. Geranium oil may ease anxiety and improve negative moods. Chamomile is calming. Kanuka oil is said to be calming and relaxing but is mostly used (like manuka oil) to treat skin problems, especially infections.

People specifically trained in aromatherapy can be found in the Yellow Pages. Alternatively, you could talk to your local chemist or find out what other people affected by dementia have found useful.

Herbal remedies

Herbal treatments include garlic, which may work by reducing cholesterol levels, ginseng, regarded as a general tonic, and gotu kola, which is reputed to improve vascular function generally, and thus increase blood supply to the brain. Ginko biloba is discussed in chapter 8. There are various other herbal and homeopathic remedies available and while they may be worth a trial, people should remember that they are not necessarily safe. Herbal remedies are not subject to the intense scrutiny applied to prescribed drugs, and may contain dangerous impurities. There is also a risk that they could interact with other medication. For example, St John's Wort interacts with some antidepressants. It is best to check with your pharmacist or doctor before taking alternative remedies by mouth.

Homeopathy

Homeopathy uses 'natural' remedies to heal people. The homeopath gives tiny doses of substances which in larger doses would cause the same symptoms as the person wants to cure, the principle being 'like cures like'. Some examples of homeopathic treatment of dementia symptoms are the use of sulphur for memory loss, especially that associated with words and names, and digitalis for difficulty in thinking or remembering.

Remedies and practitioners' names are available from health food shops. The Yellow Pages list homeopaths and suppliers of remedies. Some GPs and other mainstream health workers are also trained in this area. A Diploma in

Homeopathy has been accredited by the New Zealand Qualifications Authority, and it would be advisable to check that your homeopath has this or an equivalent recognised qualification.

Maori traditional healing

Many Maori consult traditional healers (tohunga), especially if they believe the cause of their illness is of spiritual or social origin (mate Maori). Healers may use herbal medicines, massage, interpretation of symbols and signs, and appropriate rituals. The healers are often older people with experience and understanding of peoples' relationships to each other and their environment. Traditional healers and Western-trained health professionals can work together.

Reflexology

Reflexology is a form of touch therapy that reduces stress and tension. The theory is that massaging a reflex area in the foot stimulates energy in a corresponding part of the body. Massage therapists or physiotherapists may include this among their skills. You will find reflexologists listed in the Yellow Pages.

Mainstream professional help

Occupational therapy

Occupational therapists are involved in the assessment and treatment of people with dementia. The areas of assessment involve self-care, productivity (i.e. the ability to perform paid and unpaid work) and leisure. The assessment is usually carried out in the person's home and can highlight dangers in the environment (such as rugs that an older person could slip on) and dangers from forgetfulness (pots burned dry on the stove, doors left unlocked). Occupational therapists help make the diagnosis of dementia when they assess people's level of functioning.

An occupational therapist can provide equipment and advice on how to improve a person's activities in a problem area. Some examples are:

Self-care: provision of bath boards, shower seats, advice on the best cutlery and methods of eating.

Productivity: visual cues around the kitchen; for example, labelling cupboards with their contents, reminders to turn the stove off.

Leisure: involvement in a hobby that the person can enjoy, introducing the carer to activities to share with the person with dementia; for example, hand massage, dancing.

Many occupational therapists also teach memory retraining and relaxation. In long-term care they run group activities and supervise caregivers in their quest to help the residents maintain their skills. Occupational therapists may also carry out assessments for driving safety.

Dietetics

Many people with dementia, particularly if they live alone, have a poor diet. Lack of vitamins and minerals and insufficient calorie and protein intake can cause mental functioning to deteriorate even further. Many people improve greatly once they have three square meals a day.

Late in the course of dementia, when the swallowing action deteriorates, dieticians can advise on the type and consistency of food required, and may suggest supplements (such as Complan) to maintain and equate nutrient intake. A general practitioner or hospital team can refer a patient to a dietician. Some dieticians work independently or are attached to rest homes and private hospitals. They are listed in the Yellow Pages or dietitians.org.nz/find-a-dietitian. Check first that they are interested in working with people with dementia.

Psychology

Psychologists are trained in the assessment of cognition and may be involved at the time of diagnosis (see chapter 3). Their tests give an estimate of someone's intellectual ability before the onset of their problems, so later tests can reveal whether or not there has been any deterioration. The tests they perform help identify areas of strength and weakness and this information is helpful both in making a diagnosis and planning treatment.

Psychologists often run memory retraining and cognitive behavioural therapy groups. They might be able to offer individual therapy to help the person with dementia to come to terms with the illness, or to help the family adjust to the situation. Psychologists also contribute greatly by helping carers manage behaviour that they find challenging. They are usually well trained in research methods.

Most mental health services for older people have a psychologist as part of the team. Larger centres will have private psychologists who are experienced in dementia assessment and management. Talk to your GP, someone in the public health system or Alzheimer's New Zealand to get a referral to a suitable person. You can choose a psychologist from the Yellow Pages, but when you call make sure they are interested in dementia. Get an estimate of cost first and if you have private insurance, check whether your policy covers psychology services. Neuropsychological testing takes a long time and can be expensive.

Physiotherapy

People with dementia suffer from the same physical problems as other older people. These include poor balance and falls, difficulty walking (particularly if they have suffered a stroke or have Parkinson's disease), breathing problems and pain (especially from arthritis). A physiotherapist can assess the person and provide suitable treatment. Pain is often the cause of distress or behaviour changes in people with dementia and a physiotherapist can provide non-drug relief. They often also perform alternative therapies such as acupuncture, massage and reflexology.

Physiotherapists sometimes run general exercise programmes designed to maintain people's mobility and improve their physical and mental wellbeing. These programmes can be individually tailored or done in groups.

Physiotherapists work in health services for older people, outpatient clinics and in the community. There are many private practitioners, some of whom have an interest in older people. If physiotherapy is required as the result of an accident, the Accident Compensation Corporation (ACC) may partially fund private treatment.

Social workers

Social workers are invaluable in many ways. They can put people in touch with suitable services, help arrange benefits and sort out legal matters. Sometimes they are trained in family therapy or grief counselling. Families can find them a great source of information and support. They may be attached to the public health system, residential care facilities or voluntary organisations such as Alzheimer's New Zealand or Age Concern.

Speech therapy

Speech therapists are specialists in communication and swallowing. Their assessment of language can be very helpful in diagnosing certain types of dementia. Where the diagnosis is already known, the therapist can help the person to keep talking and develop other methods of communication when speech fails. Swallowing is often a problem in the later stages of Alzheimer's disease, and may occur in vascular dementia as a result of stroke damage. The speech therapist can give advice to carers about managing eating problems. There are some private speech therapists, but most are attached to the public health system.

Miscellaneous therapies

Art therapy

The use of art can enable people whose communication is otherwise poor to express themselves. Art can be a personal statement: 'This is what my life is or has been about' or a way to release strong emotions. As people express themselves through art, they develop a relationship with the therapist or others in a group, they gain a sense of achievement and recall past accomplishments. This helps retain a sense of personal identity and self-esteem. Art therapy is useful throughout the course of dementia and the work produced may help measure the progression or stabilisation of the illness. Sometimes a person's art even improves with the development of dementia, as inhibitions are lost.

An American doctor describes the feeling in an art therapy class:

> The group seemed at ease, as if their colors and brush strokes were tapping into primitive and universal centers of their brains, capable of replacing, for the moment, their dimmed logic and language skills.[3]

Doll therapy

In doll therapy the patient, usually a woman with advanced dementia, is given a doll to look after. The woman treats the doll as a baby and can be kept occupied by dressing or 'feeding' it. Sometimes a soft toy is treated in the same way. The person often appears to be comforted by just carrying it around. This is a controversial therapy as some people see it as 'infantilising'; that is, treating the older person like a child and hence causing her to lose her dignity. On the other hand, if she enjoys the doll and is happier and calmer with it, who are we to interfere in her choice? Pragmatic people use this therapy where they find it works.

Massage

Massage can help reduce muscle tension and aid relaxation. It can be used in conjunction with aromatherapy or acupuncture. Massage therapists can visit people at home, and occasionally rest homes employ a person to give massages or to teach caregivers some basic techniques. Massage services, including some associated with particular cultures, are listed in the Yellow Pages. Make sure they offer therapeutic massage for older people (rather than the erotic type). It is helpful to ask friends or professionals for the name of a skilled massage therapist.

Music therapy

Like art, music is part of life and can be used for entertainment, relaxation or pleasure, as well as therapy. As a therapy, music can be used to promote reminiscence and discussion in a group, to allow verbal expression (through singing) when other verbal skills have gone, and to calm people or to express emotion. Often families know of a particular tune that either calmed or was enjoyed by the person with dementia. They can play this if the person is agitated or bored. Music can also make exercise regimes interesting. It is much more fun to keep up physical fitness through dance than to go through a repetitive routine in silence. Some rest homes and private hospitals employ music therapists. Like art therapists working in this area, they are few and far between.

In summary

Dementia affects different people in different ways. It is important to keep an open mind about what might help someone who has dementia, and consider their personality, previous preferences and current needs. This has been a very quick and superficial tour through some of the therapies that might be useful. The list of resources in the appendix will help you source further information.

References

[1] *Practice Guidelines for the Treatment of Psychiatric Disorders*, The American Psychiatric Association, Washington, 2000.

[2] Kitwood, Tom, *Dementia Reconsidered: The person comes first*, Open University Press, Buckingham, 1997.

[3] Firlik, Andrew D., 'A piece of my mind: Margo's logo', *Journal of the American Medical Association*, 265 (2): 201, 1991.

Chapter 8

Medical treatments for dementia

New anti-dementia compounds are very promising, but should not be prescribed without attention to individual cases. Each patient's response must be carefully monitored with regard to his or her quality of life.

STEPHEN POST [1]

This chapter is about medical treatments for dementia. Drug treatments that slow the progression of Alzheimer's disease have recently become available. There is a lot of interest and research in this area and we can expect more and better drugs to appear in the not-too-distant future. Nevertheless, treatment does not just involve the use of medication but also requires many other approaches: psychological, social and environmental, some of which were discussed in the previous chapter.

Physical or mental illness, other than dementia, can make confusion worse and needs to be treated (see chapter 3 for descriptions of delirium and depression). A sudden deterioration or change in behaviour may be caused by physical illness and the person should be checked out medically. It is important that people with dementia stay as well as possible, both physically and mentally.

Medical treatments for Alzheimer's disease

Cognition-enhancing drugs

The development of drugs called acetylcholinesterase inhibitors (ACEIs) gives new hope to people suffering from Alzheimer's disease. These are the first drugs that make a significant difference to the course of dementia. Although they were originally developed for the treatment of Alzheimer's disease, there is increasing evidence that ACEIs improve symptoms in vascular and Lewy body dementias. These drugs help about half the people who take them, but it is not yet possible to predict who will respond without a trial first.

Over the long term, the effect of this medication can wear off, and even if people remain on the optimum dose, the relentless course of dementia begins once again. Once the drugs are stopped the patient declines to the point they would have reached without treatment. This suggests that the drugs treat the symptoms of dementia but not, as far as we know, the underlying disease. We are still a long way off finding a cure.

However, even a very modest improvement in function, mood or cognitive ability can improve quality of life. Retaining a few skills that would otherwise be lost can raise the self-esteem of the person with dementia and reduce the burden on the carer. An improvement in function may extend the time a person with dementia can manage at home. These medications are worth a try.

How the ACEIs work

In chapter 2, the chemical changes occurring in the brains of people with dementia were described. In Alzheimer's disease, vascular dementia and especially Lewy body dementia, there is a shortage of the brain chemical acetylcholine (which is important in the formation of memories). Acetylcholine is broken down in the brain by the enzyme acetylcholinesterase. The ACEIs prevent acetylcholinesterase from working. The less acetylcholine that is destroyed by acetylcholinesterase, the more there is available to transmit messages around the brain and to form memories.

Butyrlcholine, a slightly different neurotransmitter, has also been found to be deficient in the brains of people with Alzheimer's disease. Some drugs also prevent butyrlcholinesterase from breaking down butyrlcholine, and raise its level as well.

The earliest ACEI was tacrine (Cognex), introduced in the early 1990s. It helped the symptoms of dementia, but caused major side effects so that most people could not tolerate the full dose. More recently, three other drugs have become available. These are: donepezil (Aricept, produced by Pfizer or *Apo-Donepezil* by Apotex NZ Ltd), rivastigmine (Exelon, produced by Novartis) and galantamine (Reminyl, produced by Janssen-Cilag). They are recommended for use in people with mild to moderate Alzheimer's disease, though it is possible they might help people even with severe dementia. They are probably most useful in Lewy body dementia and the dementia associated with Parkinson's disease.

Effectiveness

Overall, it seems that when taking ACEIs, about 40 to 50 per cent of patients show an improvement in memory, thinking or other cognitive function. Some have a reduction in the psychological problems associated with the disease (such as apathy, anxiety, depression and agitation, and an increase in wellbeing and alertness). Occasionally, people regain skills that they had lost. Often, the progression of the dementia is slowed down.

How the ACEIs are used

Doctors start patients on a low dose of the chosen ACEI, gradually increasing it to the recommended maximum. People often cannot tolerate the full, recommended dose, but may still benefit from a lower dose. The medication needs to be tried for at least three months or, better, six before deciding whether it has helped. This is because the progression of Alzheimer's disease is slow, and it takes time to tell if the drug is making any difference.

Usually patients are reviewed one month after starting treatment, to check for side effects. After three months there is a fuller assessment to decide whether the medication is helping. At this time, the doctor is likely to repeat a test of cognitive function, such as the MOCA, and ask the patient — and their family — about their ability to do their usual tasks and about any psychological or behavioural changes (for better or worse). Questionnaires or scales may be used to measure these changes. Improvements can be unexpected and hard to measure, as seen in the following situation:

> *Mr W. found that after starting on donepezil he no longer walked into things the way he used to, because he was better at judging distances. He also felt a lot better in himself. His wife reported that he seemed to be calmer and less frustrated by his memory problems. On testing there was no change in the score of his MMSE (the test measuring memory and other cognitive skills), but both Mr and Mrs W. were pleased with the slight improvement and wished to continue the treatment.*

Side effects

The side effects of the three drugs are similar, and are commonly gastric symptoms, such as loss of appetite, nausea, vomiting, diarrhoea and stomach cramps. ACEIs may worsen peptic ulcers or liver problems.

They can also slow the heart rate and aggravate existing heart problems. Dizziness, poor sleep, worsening of breathing problems and tiredness may also occur.

However, side effects are rarely severe and can usually be lessened by starting the medication at a low dose and increasing it slowly. Sometimes people take antinausea medication as well. If, for any reason, medication has to be stopped for more than a few days, it should be restarted at a lower dose to avoid side effects. ACEIs may interact with other drugs, so it is important for the prescribing doctor to know what medication the person is already taking.

Who prescribes them?

Any registered medical practitioner can prescribe these drugs. However, while some GPs will feel confident at making a diagnosis of dementia and using ACEIs, many others will wish to refer their patient to a specialist service to get a full assessment before treatment is started.

The different drugs

The main advantage of donepezil is that it is now fully subsidised by Pharmac (the government drug purchasing agency). It is thus free of charge except for dispensing fees. The usual starting dose is 5 mg a day. If this is tolerated, the dose is increased to 10 mg daily after a month. The pills come in 5- and 10-mg strengths.

Rivastigmine tablets begin at 1.5 mg twice a day, gradually working up to 6 mg twice daily. It is often difficult to achieve the maximum dose because of side effects. However, a total daily dose of 6 mg is thought to be effective. The pills come in 1.5-, 3.0-, 4.5- and 6.0-mg strengths. There is also a transdermal patch that is applied daily to the skin. This avoids many side-effects and also means the person does not have to remember several doses. The patch comes in two sizes, 5 and 10 (equivalent to 9 mg and 18 mg). Rivastigmine should not be given to people with severe liver problems. Some studies suggest that the positive effects of rivastigmine are longer lasting than those of other drugs. This could be because it acts on the enzyme butyrlcholinesterase in addition to acetylcholinesterase.

The long-acting form of galantamine is taken daily, the dose beginning at 8 mg and increasing to 16 mg daily after four weeks. The maximum recommended dose is 24 mg daily. Galantamine works on another neurotransmitter system, the nicotinic system, as well as the acetylcholine system. People with severe liver or kidney problems should not take galantamine.

The cost to the patient of a month's supply of these medicines (other than the generic brand of donepezil, which is funded) is $130–$250, depending on the chemist. Each drug company provides a free starter pack for the first month. This means that people can try the drug to make sure they don't get major side effects before they commit to any ongoing expense.

How long to stay on them?

In the UK, the government pays for these drugs for as long as the person is getting some benefit from them. If their MMSE score falls below 12, or if the person is placed in residential care, the situation must be reviewed to ensure that the drugs are still beneficial. If people are still being helped in some way, for example, by staying calmer or having less trouble with hallucinations, then doctors continue to prescribe the medication.

In New Zealand, there are no official restrictions on how long someone should stay on ACEIs. However, for people who clearly do not benefit, there is little point in continuing with the medication. In other cases, it is hard to tell whether the drugs are actually making much difference in slowing the progression of the disease. One way to decide this is to have a brief medication-free trial. Someone who rapidly gets worse when taken off the drug was probably benefiting from it; if there is no noticeable change, they could probably do without it. One of the problems with this approach is that if people deteriorate in the drug-free period, then when treatment is restarted, they do not always get back to the level they were at before stopping the drug. If the effect of the first drug wears off, it might be worth swapping to another ACEI. (This makes sense, bearing in mind their slightly different types of action.) We do not know yet which might be the best drug to start on in any individual case, but this is something that might become clearer in the future. Usually, people are started on donepezil because, since coming off patent, Pharmac is funding it.

Financial cost

ACEI therapy, other than with donepezil, incurs a significant cost to individuals; about $3000 per year and this could continue for many years. Some people can afford this and are willing to pay for anything that might help. Sometimes the family will chip in.

People with a Community Services Card may be eligible for a disability allowance from Work and Income New Zealand (WINZ) to help pay for the medication. To qualify for funding people need to have:

- An annual income of less than a particular specified amount.
- A letter from the doctor stating that there is no other medication suitable for you.

WINZ can pay up to a maximum amount of $60.17 per week (in 2012) towards the expenses incurred in paying for medication. If the person is already receiving some disability allowance funds (for example, costs of doctor's visits or transport), then this amount is subtracted from the total and there will be less available to pay for medication. An application for disability allowance needs to be filled in, together with an income and asset declaration; both forms are obtained from WINZ. A social worker or a person from Alzheimer's New Zealand can help with the paperwork if necessary.

See www.workandincome.govt.nz/individuals/a-z-benefits/disability-allowance.html

Ethical problems

Dementia is a progressive condition, and people with dementia and their families work through certain crises and adapt to each new level of disability as it surfaces. If someone's ability improves with medication, this is usually only temporary and when they deteriorate, the crisis has to be worked through again. This just repeats the distress already experienced. One of the saddest outcomes of ACEI therapy can be that a person regains their insight and realises once more that there is something wrong with them.

> *One of my patients who had Alzheimer's disease cheerfully denied there was anything wrong with her and carried on her life in a small, tolerant community while her daughter gradually took over her affairs.*
>
> *After a while on donepezil she came in for a review. She looked anxious and perplexed and struggled to explain herself. 'I'm . . . I'm . . . not there . . .' she said, having now realised something was wrong. I doubted that I had done her any favours with the treatment.*

Supervision of medication

It can be hard to ensure that people living on their own take their medication correctly. They may forget to take their pill altogether, or forget that they have already taken one and so take another. The family or other carers have to supervise the taking of medication and this can involve extra work. The use of patches can reduce the need for so much supervision.

Is it worth it?

Whether or not drug treatment is right for any one patient comes down to a question of cost versus benefit. Are the side effects, the risk of increasing distress and hassle of having to remember to take the pills worth the possibility of some benefit? Taking the medication for a trial period could help to decide this.

Some people accept their own or a relative's dementia and wish to let nature take its course. Others want to do everything within their power to retain the person's abilities for as long as possible, despite the downsides of treatment.

Other medical treatments

Many of the following treatments have not been proven to work in scientific trials. However, there is some theoretical evidence that they should work and some individuals report a good response. If they do not have serious side effects, it may be worth giving them a trial.

Memantine

Glutamic acid is a compound that damages brain cells. It is released after injury, such as that caused by the loss of blood supply or Alzheimer's disease. A drug called memantine (Ebixa), produced by Lundbeck in New Zealand, prevents the release of glutamic acid and so reduces the amount of damage. Memantine has been shown to be effective in slowing the rate of progression of even severe dementia in some cases. Side effects include hallucinations, confusion, headaches, dizziness and tiredness. The dose is gradually increased to 10 mg twice daily. It costs about the same as the ACEIs and is not funded by Pharmac.

Antioxidants

As we age, we accumulate free radicals (a form of oxygen) which cause the damage associated with growing old. It is thought that free radicals in the brain may cause or contribute to cell death in dementia. Antioxidants soak up these free radicals and prevent damage being done to nerve cells. Some studies have indicated that antioxidants slow the progress of Alzheimer's disease, though others have not shown any particular benefit.

The best-known antioxidant is Vitamin E (alpha-tocopherol). The American Psychiatric Association recommends a dose of 200–800 IU (International Units) per day (about half a cup of blueberries). There are few side effects, but inflammation of the veins (thrombophlebitis) has been reported and there may be some detrimental interaction with blood-thinning agents such as warfarin. Other antioxidants are Vitamin C and green tea.

The drug selegiline, usually prescribed for Parkinson's disease, is also an antioxidant and some studies have suggested it improves cognitive function. However, there are side effects, including the potential to interact with other prescribed drugs, and it is not recommended yet as treatment for dementia.

Ginko biloba

Ginko biloba is an extract from the leaves of a Chinese tree. It increases the blood supply to the brain, prevents blood clotting (avoiding strokes) and helps brain cells withstand poor oxygen supply. Its main action, however, may be as an antioxidant.

In the one major study, ginko appeared to stabilise and occasionally improve patients with dementia compared to those who were untreated. Other studies have shown some mild positive effects. Some individuals find ginko very helpful. There do not seem to be any major side effects, but it should be used cautiously in people who bleed easily or who are already on medication to prevent clotting, such as warfarin or aspirin. The recommended dose is 120–240 mg daily.[2] It comes in a variety of forms and can be bought at health food shops and pharmacies.

Anti-inflammatory drugs

In Alzheimer's disease the brain responds to some of the physical changes, such as the formation of plaques and tangles, by becoming inflamed, which causes further damage. Anti-inflammatory drugs reduce the inflammatory response and limit the amount of damage. These drugs are often used for arthritis and there is some evidence to suggest that people who have taken anti-inflammatories for a long time earlier in life are less prone to getting Alzheimer's disease. However, it has not been shown that they help once Alzheimer's disease has started. These drugs cause side effects in older people that can be quite dangerous, such as stomach ulcers and bleeding. Some of the newer anti-inflammatories, such as the COX-2 inhibitors, cause fewer gastric problems but may affect the heart.

Oestrogen

Some studies have shown that oestrogen, used as hormone replacement after menopause, cuts the incidence of Alzheimer's disease. However, women who take oestrogen are generally more health conscious and better educated than average. General good health and education in themselves protect against Alzheimer's disease, so it is not clear what is doing the work here. Other studies suggest oestrogen might increase the risk of Alzheimer's. There is nothing to suggest that giving oestrogen to someone who has already developed Alzheimer's disease is helpful.

Recent research suggests that oestrogen use over the long term can be dangerous, increasing the risk of some cancers and heart attacks. As the evidence for oestrogen helping in Alzheimer's disease is not convincing, the risks appear to outweigh any possible advantages.

Statins

Statins are drugs that are used to reduce cholesterol levels. They may help prevent Alzheimer's disease, and further trials are planned to assess this.

Treatments for non-Alzheimer's dementias

Vascular dementia

Treatments to preserve blood vessels

The treatment for vascular dementia involves much the same strategies as used in preventing the onset of the disease:

- *High blood pressure* should be brought back to normal. (Reducing blood pressure also seems to prevent Alzheimer's disease.)
- *Lowering blood cholesterol* levels helps to keep damage to arteries to a minimum and ultimately reduces the risk of stroke. Cholesterol levels are reduced by adjusting diet or the use of statin drugs.
- *Stopping smoking* may help to prevent further damage to blood vessels and so limit the amount of brain damage caused by a reduction in blood flow.
- A small dose of *aspirin* (75–150 mg, $^{1}/_{4}$–$^{1}/_{2}$ of a tablet per day) prevents clotting in the blood vessels of the brain and may slow the progress of vascular dementia. Specially coated tablets that do not irritate the stomach are available. People who cannot take aspirin may be prescribed dipyridamole (Persantin).
- Sometimes blood clots form in the heart or in the carotid arteries in the neck. Surgery on narrowed carotid arteries can reduce the chance of a clot forming, then breaking off and travelling to the brain. An anticoagulant, warfarin, is prescribed if problems with the heart mean that clots could develop there, then go to the brain.

Folic acid

Homocysteine, a by-product of many bodily reactions, is found in higher levels in vascular dementia (and also Alzheimer's disease). Folic acid, normally prescribed at a dose of 5 mg daily, reduces the level of homocysteine and may slow progression of both disorders.

Acetylcholinesterase inhibitors

Recent research on the use of donepezil, rivastigmine and galantamine suggests that the ACEIs are all effective in slowing the course of vascular dementia. This is not surprising as the end result of cell death, from whatever cause, is a drop in the level of acetylcholine. (Memantine has also been shown to be useful.)

Mixed dementia

All the strategies used for Alzheimer's disease and vascular dementia can be tried to treat mixed dementia.

Lewy body dementia

In Lewy body dementia, the drop in level of acetylcholine is severe. ACEIs may be even more helpful in Lewy body dementia than in Alzheimer's disease. These drugs improve attention and may also help ameliorate psychotic symptoms such as hallucinations. There are varying reports on whether they help or hinder Parkinson's-like symptoms.

It may be worth trying any of the strategies listed for the other dementias, with the exception of selegiline, which can worsen hallucinations.

Frontotemporal dementia

In these dementias no abnormalities have been found in the acetylcholine system, so it is unsurprising that the sufferers do not benefit from the use of ACEIs.

However, some abnormal behaviour, such as poor self-control, overeating and repetitive (compulsive) actions respond to selective serotonin re-uptake inhibitors (SSRIs), a form of antidepressant. The SSRIs available in New Zealand are fluoxetine (Prozac), paroxetine (Aropax), citalopram (Cipramil), escitalopram (Lexapro) and sertraline (Arrow-Sertraline).

In summary

For many people the new anti-dementia drugs will either slow the speed of progression of dementia or cause improvement. They have side effects, though, and it takes time to see whether the beneficial effects outweigh the disadvantages. Whether to use such medication is something patients and their families have to decide, along with their doctor. Research in this area is ongoing and more effective, safer medications may be available shortly.

People with dementia need to keep in optimum health and use non-medical approaches to their care, as well as drugs. Some treatments help some people but not others. It is worth patiently working through the options.

References

[1] Post, Stephen G., 'The fear of forgetfulness: A grassroots approach to an ethics of Alzheimer's disease', *The Journal of Clinical Ethics*, 9 (1):75, 1998.

[2] Jones, Roy, *Drug Treatment in Dementia*, Blackwell Science, Oxford, 2000.

Chapter 9

Behavioural and psychological difficulties

In reality we cannot change a person, but we can influence their behaviour by how we respond to it and by being aware of our own behaviours when we feel under pressure. The actions we take are the key.

SIGN IN THE NURSES' OFFICE AT PUKEKOHE HOSPITAL

Emotional disturbances and behaviour that create challenges in care occur commonly in people with dementia. This chapter aims to help the reader understand the complex interaction between the person, the dementing illness, physical factors and the care environment. If we are able to understand the causes of challenging behaviour, we are able to think of solutions.

During the course of dementia 70–80 per cent of people will show some sort of 'challenging' behaviour. Most people become depressed or anxious at some point. Psychotic symptoms, such as hallucinations (perceiving things that are not there) and delusions (false beliefs), occur in at least 50 per cent of people with dementia.

Different problems surface at different stages. For example, depression, perhaps a response to the awareness that things are not right, occurs in the earlier stages of Alzheimer's disease, but wears off as the illness develops. More severe behaviour disturbances are most likely to surface when a person's ability to talk has diminished and behavioural expression is the only way to communicate, that is, when the dementia is moderately advanced.

Different types of dementia cause different problems. For example, in frontotemporal dementia there may be poor control of sexual impulses. Hallucinations are common in Lewy body dementia.

These disturbances are sometimes the reason that care at home becomes impossible. However, often the behaviour is not risky and does not distress the person with dementia. In these cases the caregiver may need to just accept and tolerate the behaviour or make simple changes to routines to accommodate it. It is important to remember that many so-called 'challenging' or 'problem' behaviours are of no concern at all to the person with dementia. The challenge is for the caregiver to cope with them.

Types of problems

Psychological/psychiatric problems

Some of the more common psychological symptoms of dementia are:

- Anxiety, panic attacks, repeated actions, often to reassure the person (these occur in up to 40 per cent of cases of dementia)
- Depression (20–40 per cent)
- Hallucinations/misinterpreting sights or sounds (more than 30 per cent)
- Paranoia or other delusions, i.e. false beliefs (30 per cent)
- Loss of emotional control, 'lability' (weeping, laughing, becoming angry at very little or at the wrong time).

Behavioural problems

Some sorts of behaviour which cause concern are:

- Agitation (restlessness with anxiety)
- Aggression, such as yelling abuse or hitting out
- Apathy, lack of motivation and inactivity, withdrawal from company
- Calling out for no obvious reason
- Clinging behaviour: this is also called 'shadowing' or 'trailing', i.e. following someone around closely and not letting them out of sight
- Hoarding: the person saves up rubbish or collects various useless items
- Losing bladder or bowel control, or urinating or passing bowel motions in unsuitable places
- Repetitive behaviour, such as doing or saying things over and over again (especially repeating questions)
- Resisting care, that is, not cooperating or fighting off helpers
- Sexually inappropriate behaviour: this could be lewd comments, touching others in a sexual way or masturbating in public
- Sleep disturbances (too little, too much, at the wrong time)
- Undressing in public
- Wandering, pacing endlessly or actively escaping.

People often display more than one problem behaviour, and behavioural and psychological problems overlap. Psychological problems can cause a change in behaviour, and unusual behaviour may incur a negative response from others, which distresses the person with dementia. A physical change in the brain or body is often the reason for a sudden change in emotions and behaviour.

Causes of behavioural and psychological problems

There is usually no easy answer to the question 'what is causing this problem?', because often there are many issues to consider.

Challenging behaviour is the outcome of interactions between some or all of the following factors:

- The usual personality of the person with dementia
- Their lifetime experiences (past history) and habits
- The damage done to the brain by the illness
- Their current social, physical and emotional environment
- Responses to the behaviour.

Taking these factors one at a time, it is sometimes possible to predict certain behaviours in a particular situation.

Personality

Personality is the way we typically think about ourselves and other people. It determines the way we interact with others and shapes how we characteristically respond to what is going on around us. An individual's personality will make a difference to how they cope with the changes occurring in dementia. For example:

- A woman who is usually placid becomes apathetic when she develops dementia;
- A wife who has always been anxious does not let her husband out of her sight (shadowing);
- A man who was normally suspicious and mistrustful becomes paranoid as his faculties deteriorate.

Mr G. had always been an independent loner who responded to people interfering in his life with verbal and sometimes physical abuse. He was very controlling and had often been violent towards his family.

It came as no surprise that when a series of strokes affected his memory, speech and balance, his usual response to nursing care was to hit out at the staff.

Although previous personality is important, we need to remember that all forms of dementia (but particularly those affecting the frontal lobes) can affect personality, so that people do not react as they might have before their illness.

Personal experiences

It is easy to see how a person's life experience will interact with their present situation. (This is sometimes difficult to disentangle from personality, as experience affects the development of personality. Also, a particular personality style will result in certain life experiences.)

The following are some examples of past history affecting behaviour when a person develops dementia:

- Someone who has experienced nurturing and kindness will find it easier to accept being dependent on others and will be less likely to be difficult with caregivers.
- A person who has previously been sexually abused is likely to respond to personal care involving the removal of clothes (such as for showering or toileting) with fear, resistance or physical aggression.

Mr H. spent several years in the 1940s as a Japanese prisoner of war. When he was admitted to a locked hospital ward he became very agitated and constantly attempted to leave. It was very difficult to reassure him that our aim was to help him rather than administer any sort of punishment or torture.

Brain damage

Damage to certain areas of the brain will produce specific emotional or behaviour changes in anyone. Frontal lobe damage can make it difficult for a person to be aware of social niceties or can make them apathetic and lacking in motivation. Stroke damage to a specific region of the frontal lobe often results in depression. Temporal lobe injury can cause unprovoked aggression or hallucinations. Other specific changes, such as the loss of ability to recognise faces (controlled by the parietal and occipital lobes), can cause difficulty if a person does not recognise their family and caregivers and rejects them. People who have lost their sense of direction (controlled by the parietal lobe) often get lost.

Mr J., who has Alzheimer's disease, no longer recognises his house as his own and is angry with his wife for buying this new one without his involvement. Some evenings, he packs up his possessions and is ready to leave to go back to his real home. Mrs J. persuades him to come out with her for a drive and usually when they get back he accepts that this place will be OK to stay at for the night.

Loss of speech, as the result of dementia, is a major contributor to behavioural change. As verbal skills are lost, people with dementia have to rely more and more on behaviour to express their needs. Carers can learn to interpret the meaning of behaviours and emotions in the person who has lost speech. Examples of behavioural and emotional expressions of needs are:

- A woman pulls up her skirt when she wants to go to the toilet.
- A man becomes irritable and abusive when he is in pain.

Current environment

Generally, people with dementia cope better in their own home, for it is a familiar living environment. Here they know where things are and can find their way around. With a change in living circumstances (such as going into respite care) people with dementia have to adapt to changes in noise levels, access to the outside and the location of the toilet among other things. The change in physical environment will increase their confusion and lead to changes in behaviour.

The personal physical environment incorporates the person's bodily health. Many unwelcome psychological or behavioural changes are caused by medical or psychiatric illness or side effects of medication.

The social environment (such as a hospital) may subject the patient to institutional practices (such as requiring a certain level of cleanliness) that can provoke resistance and hostility. A person with dementia may find it hard to adjust to even a minor change in routine, and will express this by behaving in an unusual way. A change in caregiver, even without a change in place or routine, can also be difficult for the person to accept.

There is also an emotional environment, to which people with failing cognitive abilities can be acutely sensitive. If they detect disapproval they may become anxious and lose confidence. Fearfulness on the carer's part may communicate itself to the person with dementia, who then also becomes frightened and may act in accordance with this fear.

In the following example, a man with dementia was aware of sadness:

While she was caring for her husband with Alzheimer's disease, Mrs K.'s mother died. Mr K. did not seem to take in that his mother-in-law had died, but was aware of his wife's grief. He started to 'shadow' her, staying very close, even following her to the toilet.

Mrs K. believed that he was trying to comfort and protect her, but she felt desperate for a little solitude so that she could properly mourn the loss of her mother.

Responses to the behaviour

The way people respond to a behaviour can change it for better or worse.

- A woman trails her husband closely. If 'told off' or ignored, she becomes more anxious. On the other hand, reassuring her that she is loved and will not be abandoned helps, at least temporarily.
- A man in a rest home, when bored, pushes the person sitting next to him. The caregivers respond by rushing up and telling him to stop. This has the effect of entertaining him, so he pushes others to get the same result.
- A man becomes agitated and paces around at mealtimes, becoming angry when told to sit down. The staff realise that the bustle in the dining room is upsetting him and allow him to eat by himself in a quiet room.

Some responses to difficult behaviour can convert one problem into another, possibly worse, one. Medication is often used to control challenging behaviour, but there is a downside as most drugs have unwanted side effects to which people with dementia are especially sensitive. Giving a tranquilliser can make an alert person who is calling out so drowsy that they can no longer stand or cooperate with care. Other responses create even greater problems, as shown in the following example:

Mrs L., a frail lady with advanced dementia, lived in a private hospital. She wandered constantly and sometimes tripped. The nurses could not keep as close a watch on her as they wished and feared that in the next fall she would break her hip. Her family gave permission to restrain Mrs L. in her chair for brief periods when the staff were likely to be distracted (such as mealtimes).

Mrs L., however, became extremely agitated when her movements were restricted and fought so hard to get out of the chair that she often bruised or tore her fragile skin.

The family and staff then agreed that it was better to let her room. They preferred to accept the risk of her falling than the certain distress and injury associated with her being restrained in her chair. They bought a set of hip protectors to try to reduce the risk of a fracture.

Dealing with problem behaviours

Is it really a problem?

The first step is to decide whether the behavioural or psychological symptom really is a problem that needs attention or whether it is of little or no consequence. Hallucinations, for example, might or might not matter. Often people with dementia, especially those who live alone, see other people around them: relatives, children coming in to play, people sitting in the garden. Responses to these hallucinations vary. Some people enjoy the company, even going to the extent of preparing food for their 'visitors', but others become angry and want to chase the intruders out. There seems little harm in allowing an old lady to talk to her long-dead sister whom she sees sitting in the living room. (It may even be beneficial for her to express herself in this way.) On the other hand, an agitated man who is threatening non-existent people in his backyard may damage the garden, himself or others who get in his way. (Hallucinations are often associated with delirium, so if they begin abruptly or are associated with signs of delirium the person should be checked out by a GP.)

Another 'non-problem' might be 'pacing' by someone who has always been active and is used to walking around while solving problems. Does it matter if an old man urinates in the garden or mistakes his caregiver for a daughter and tries to kiss her? Often all that is needed is the understanding that these things are part of the condition and not deliberate antisocial acts. While such behaviour is probably not 'normal' by usual standards, this does not necessarily mean that it has to change.

Mrs L. had an old photograph of her husband propped up on the pillow in her bed. She believed that the photo was her husband, who had died many years before and seemed to enjoy having him there. Occasionally she decided to feed him. This made a mess of the sheets, so the family had to wash them more often than usual, but otherwise there were no major negative effects from Mrs L.'s misinterpretation.

A behaviour may be a problem in one setting but not another. For example, a man's repetitive questioning or 'shadowing' may be very stressful for a 24-hour-a-day caregiver wife, but if a professional worker at a day-care centre becomes impatient with him, they can ask another carer to look after him. A man may take his clothes off in his own living room if he wants, but if he removes them at the bowling club, that is another matter.

A behaviour can also be a problem at some times and not others. After a sleepless night, a caregiver may find that a behaviour she usually ignores has suddenly become intensely irritating. (The issue to be addressed here is the sleepless night, not the behaviour that has become irritating.)

Whose problem is it?

A person with dementia does not exist in a vacuum. Family and professional carers, fellow residents in a rest home, or companions at clubs or day care may all be affected by a particular behaviour. It is sometimes difficult to decide whose needs take preference. However, as people with dementia are limited in their ability to change, it is usually those around them who have to adapt.

Attempting to change behaviour which distresses caregivers will not necessarily help the person with dementia. Apathy in previously active people understandably upsets family members. However, it does not always bother people with dementia, and when attempts are made to get them out and doing things, they can become distressed. Most of us think that doing things is better than just sitting around, but this may not be true for a particular individual with dementia. The following is an example of a behaviour that was a problem for nurses but not the person with dementia.

> *The nurses in a general hospital asked for help in managing a woman who called out all day, but could not tell nurses what she wanted when they went to her. Numerous possible causes, such as pain or a full bladder, were considered, but no reason for her calling out was found. The nurses felt upset that they couldn't seem to help her.*
>
> *After observing her for a while, it became obvious that she called out whenever anyone came into her field of vision. The sound she was making was a greeting rather than a request for anything.*
>
> *This information was relayed to the nurses, who then responded by returning her greeting as they passed. There was no change in the calling out, but it ceased to be a problem.*

Family members and staff are often aghast when a couple in residential care, both with dementia (and not married to each other), get involved in an intimate relationship. If both people with dementia seem to be enjoying the relationship, who has the problem? If children find such behaviour difficult to cope with, they could talk things over with their GP or a counsellor.

Sometimes others have no difficulty coping with unusual behaviour, but the person with dementia does. In this case they need treatment or help coming to terms with the situation as in the following example.

> *A retired businessman with vascular dementia found that when he meant to laugh, he cried. He was also much more inclined to cry over the slightest thing, though he did not have other symptoms of depression.*
>
> *His wife and friends understood that this was the lability associated with dementia and accepted the increased and somewhat unusual emotional expression. However, he was embarrassed by his poor emotional control and wanted something done about it.*

There are obviously times when a particular behaviour (which does not bother the person with dementia) cannot just be accepted or ignored. If it is upsetting others or is dangerous, such as punching caregivers or frightening fellow residents, then the problem needs to be dealt with. The first step is to try to work out why the behaviour is occurring.

Working out what is happening

As discussed above, people's personalities, experiences, degree of dementia, physical condition and the environment affect behaviour. Working out why a particular behaviour is being exhibited is a five-step process.

Gathering information

The person with dementia may be able to answer simple questions such as, 'Are you in pain?' 'Are you frightened?' Discussions with people who know the person with dementia well can produce some clues: 'She's always like this when she has a bladder infection . . .', 'It started after we changed the furniture around . . .'.

Careful observation can also clarify what is happening. It helps to describe in detail what the actual behaviour is. For example, rather than 'wandering', an ex-farmer is noted to be 'walking round the rest home trying to open locked doors and windows, saying the cows need milking'. When does this happen? What was he doing when the behaviour started? Who was with him? How did people around him respond? What happened afterwards? What seemed to settle things down? By asking these sorts of questions you can get a clearer picture of what is troubling the person.

Deciding what is wrong

How do we decide what is actually happening when there are many possible options? It is useful to try to understand the person's behaviour in the context of their past habits or personality. Everyone involved with the person — their family, friends, paid caregivers and professionals — should be looking for answers. The family can share information that professional caregivers need; for example, they may reveal that the person with dementia has always been modest and is therefore unlikely to cooperate when bathed. Sometimes inspired guesswork, based on past knowledge of the person, gives us the answer. There may be surprising reasons for a person to behave in an unusual manner; for example, their caregiver may look like or have a similar manner to their bossy elder sister. It took me a while to work out what was happening with a man I was supposed to be helping:

> *A private hospital resident always seemed to get more agitated when I came to see him. After a few visits the family mentioned that he hated to see women dressed in red — 'the devil's colour'. Subsequently, I toned down my outfit on the days I knew I was going to meet him so that my time with him was more productive.*

Working through a checklist

If someone can't explain what is happening and there is no obvious answer, look through this checklist. Could the cause be:

Medical:

- Infection or other illness
- Pain or other discomfort (don't forget dental problems)
- Constipation
- A drug reaction
- Poor mobility (leading to frustration)
- Itchiness, shortness of breath or nausea
- Reduced vision or poor hearing (have they lost their glasses or hearing aid?).

Psychological:

- Depression
- Anxiety
- Psychosis (hallucinations or delusions).

Other physical problems:

- Too cold or too hot
- Hungry
- Thirsty
- Tired
- Uncomfortable (does the patient have a full bladder or bowel?).

Environmental:

- Too much or too little stimulation
- Too much noise
- A tense atmosphere because of family strife or other emotional issues
- Other residents in care who are disturbing the person or invading their space
- Poor communication: the carers don't understand what the person is trying to tell them
- 'Sundowning', i.e. agitation and restlessness at the end of the day.

Changing places

Put yourself in the shoes of the person with dementia. How would you feel if . . .

- You had to sit around all day doing nothing?
- You couldn't find the toilet and you needed to go?
- You couldn't see what was happening and someone came and tried to move you somewhere else and you didn't know why?
- You expected the children back from school any minute and were locked up in this place and couldn't get home?

It doesn't take much imagination to realise that you would cause a disturbance to break the boredom, wet yourself or urinate in the wrong place, resist the people attempting to care for you or try desperately to get out. Putting yourself in the place of the patient can give you an idea of what is wrong and how to deal with it.

Solutions for problem behaviours

After deciding what might be causing the problem it is a matter of trying some solutions to see if they help. Given the opportunity, family members and carers often come up with creative ideas to deal with the problem. Even if they do not hit on the right solution first time, something has been learned, and they know not to try that again. This is a laborious process but will help to eventually clarify what is actually happening. Sometimes carers feel desperate for a quick solution. Unfortunately, a methodical process of trial and error is usually necessary.

The sorts of possible solutions are environmental, behavioural and chemical.

Some environmental solutions

- Establish a routine that suits the person with dementia; for example, let them lie in late in the morning if that's what they like, or allow them to get up at 5 a.m. if they are naturally an early riser.
- Arrange the living situation to suit the patient; for example, make sure there is a safe outdoor area for them to walk if they hate to be inside.
- Make specific environmental adjustments, such as changing the lock on the door if a patient wanders into the street at night.
- Try to do a task later if the person resists your first attempts.

Some possible behavioural solutions

- Tolerate the behaviour (avoid arguing or scolding).
- Ignore unwanted behaviour or walk away. Be positive and praise the person for doing something more suitable.
- Distract the person. Try to focus their attention away from the event that is upsetting them (providing a cup of tea has saved many difficult situations).
- Use empathy and humour to diffuse tension.
- Maintain respect and do not treat people with dementia as naughty children. They will pick up on insults.
- Don't say to the person, 'I just told you that'. They will have forgotten what you said but will detect the tone of exasperation in your voice.
- Slow the pace of your actions and avoid rushing the patient. It can be very frightening to be rushed off to an unknown place.
- Repeat explanations and reassure the patient frequently.
- Communicate clearly, using eye contact, gestures and touch. Give simple directions, one at a time. (See more about this in chapter 6, Communication.)
- Break tasks down into small steps.

Some chemical (medical) solutions

- Treat any underlying medical conditions.
- Treat any underlying psychiatric conditions.

(Adapted from *Guidelines for the Support and Management of People with Dementia*, National Advisory Committee on Health and Disability/ADARDS, 1997.)

SOLUTIONS FOR SPECIFIC PROBLEMS

Problem	**Possible solution**
Medical	
Infection or other illness	*Make appointment with GP, treat illness*
Pain (from known cause)	*Administer regular pain relief (don't wait until the person becomes distressed)*
Constipation	*Administer fluids (or ice blocks to suck), fruit, kiwifruit juice, talk to nurse or GP*
Drug reactions	*Check with the prescriber before stopping medication*
Poor mobility	*Arrange for physiotherapy; walking aids may be required*
Other forms of discomfort	*Check with doctor*
Poor vision and hearing	*Get hearing aid tested, clean glasses, use different form of communication (such as writing or gestures)*
Psychological	
Depression	*Increase activities, encourage family visits; give counselling to help person adapt to changes; medication may be needed*
Anxiety	*Look at sources of their worry, explain frequently what is happening, try to give the person control, make things as predictable as possible, avoid known triggers for anxiety, use distraction and calming music*
Psychosis	*Ignore if not upsetting, reassure, gently explain the reality, treat with medication*

Other Physical	
Too cold or too hot	*Use thermostat-controlled heating (that can't be turned off by the frugal older person), check for multiple layers of clothing; experiment to find the best temperature*
Hungry or thirsty	*People who pace get hungry and can be provided with finger food (such as sandwiches) to eat on the go; food supplements such as Complan are ideal for people who have trouble eating*
Tiredness	*Prevent afternoon irritability by ensuring a nap after lunch, avoid difficult tasks (such as showering) when patient is tired*
Full bladder or bowel	*Take person to the toilet regularly, learn to read signs, e.g. fiddling with trousers*
Environmental	
Noise	*Ensure patient has a quiet place to go to, avoid leaving them in noisy areas (like dining rooms in residential care)*
Too much stimulation	*Avoid too much confusing activity and noise, keep groups of visitors small; at family gatherings keep the person in a quiet area where they can have one-to-one conversations; turn off background noises such as TV*
Too little stimulation	*Encourage person to attend groups, play their favourite music, videos, walk, sit outside, adapt previous activities (e.g. the housewife can fold towels, the gardener can do some weeding)*
Tense atmosphere	*Argue out of the sight and earshot of the person with dementia; get counselling help for unfinished family business that interferes*

	with caregiving; try to agree on a consistent approach to challenging problem behaviours
Other residents	*Discuss with the residential-care manager if other residents upset the person with dementia*
Poor communication	*Explain things simply and repeat explanations often*
Sundowning	*Get person to rest after lunch and take an evening walk*

Psychiatric drugs

The behaviour problems associated with dementia can be frightening, frustrating or dangerous. Caregivers (professional or family) often only seek help when they are at the end of their tether and want something done immediately. Medication appears to be a quick fix, but drugs can cause side effects that make the person less able to function and make it more difficult to find the cause of the problem.

In the past, and probably still, drugs were used excessively to treat difficult behaviour. Hopefully, as understanding of dementia improves, clinicians will be less inclined to reach for the prescription pad. Now that we recognise these behaviours are often an attempt to communicate, we should try to work out what people with dementia are trying to say, rather than trying to stop them saying it.

Medication should be used only after carefully evaluating the situation and trying behavioural approaches or environmental changes to resolve the problem. If the underlying problem causing challenging behaviour is one that is known to respond to drug treatment (e.g. psychosis), psychiatric medication is quite appropriate. Anti-dementia drugs are sometimes helpful in managing the behaviour difficulties associated with dementia. There are some circumstances when using medication is the only humane response; for example, when a person is very upset and environmental and behavioural changes have not helped overcome this.

Drugs that are used in this area are listed below.

Name of drug (most common)	**Use**	**Daily dose** (range mg)	**Side effects** (most common)
Antipsychotics *			
Newer types			
Risperidone (Risperdal)	*Psychosis, agitation, aggression*	*0.25–2.0*	*Extrapyramidal symptoms (EPSE)† headache, low BP‡*

Olanzapine§ (Zyprexa)	*Psychosis, agitation, aggression*	*2.5–5.0*	*Weight gain, sleepiness, low BP‡*
Quetiapine§ (Seroquel)	*Psychosis, agitation, aggression*	*12.5–100.0+*	*Sleepiness*
Older types			
Haloperidol (Serenace)	*Psychosis, agitation, aggression*	*0.25–3.0*	*EPSE†*
Pericyazine (Neulactil)	*Psychosis, agitation, aggression*	*2.5–10.0*	*EPSE†, sedation*
Thioridazine (Melleril)	*Psychosis, agitation, aggression, anxiety*	*10–75.0*	*Low BP‡, heart irregularities*
Anti-anxiety			
Benzodiazepines: diazepam, lorazepam, clonazepam	*Anxiety, agitation*	*Varies*	*Sedation, falls, confusion, memory loss, dependence on the medication¤*
Buspirone (Buspar, Biron)	*Anxiety, agitation*	*5–30.0*	*Headache, dizziness*
Hypnotics			
Benzodiazepines: temazepam, triazolam, lormetazepam	*To aid sleep*	*Varies*	*Falls, confusion, memory loss, dependence, daytime sleepiness*
Zopiclone (Imovane)	*To aid sleep*	*3.75–15.0*	*Bad taste, daytime sleepiness*
Antidepressants †			
Paroxetine (Aropax)	*Improve mood, reduce anxiety and aggression, stop repetitive behaviour*	*10–50.0*	*Nausea, drowsiness, low blood sodium levels*
Citalopram (Cipramil)	*Improve mood, reduce anxiety and aggression, stop repetitive behaviour*	*10–40.0*	*Nausea, drowsiness, low blood sodium levels*
Tricyclics			
Nortriptyline, clomipramine	*Improve mood, reduce anxiety and aggression, stop repetitive behaviour*	*Varies*	*Many and varied*

Anticonvulsants (mood stabilisers)			
Carbamazepine§ (Tegretol)	*Reduce aggression and impulsive behaviour*	*50–200+*	*Sleepiness, confusion, blood and liver problems*
Sodium valproate§ (Epilim)	*Reduce aggression and impulsive behaviour*	*200+*	*Gait and balance problems, nausea, blood changes, weight gain*
Others			
Cyproterone (Androcur)	*Reduce sex drive*	*50–100*	*Liver problems, breast enlargement*
Cholinesterase inhibitors and memantine	*May reduce problems generally*	*Varies*	*Nausea*

**All antipsychotics may slightly increase the risk of stroke when used in dementia.*
† Extrapyramidal side effects (EPSE) are symptoms similar to Parkinson's disease, such as shaking, stiffness, changes in walking, dribbling, loss of facial expression. There are other medications to get rid of these side effects (e.g. benztropine), but they cause problems of their own (like increased confusion).
‡ Low blood pressure (BP). If blood pressure drops too low people can become dizzy, unsteady on their feet and may fall. Often blood pressure can drop suddenly when a person stands up.
§ Not currently approved for this use by Pharmac.
¤ Dependence means a person cannot stop using a drug without getting withdrawal symptoms (for benzodiazepines, these are increased anxiety and agitation, shakes, confusion). They may need to keep on increasing the dose to obtain the same effect.
† Fluoxetine (Prozac) is less suitable for older people because it interacts with other drugs and is very long acting, so if there are side effects they take a long while to disappear once the drug is stopped.

Medication should usually be used for only a short time before attempts are made to withdraw it. (In Australia it is mandatory for doctors to review every month the medication used for the behavioural symptoms of dementia.) This helps avoid long-term side effects as well as checking whether the drug is still needed. As the dementia progresses, or as changes are made in the environment, the behaviour of concern may disappear and medication can be stopped. Many residential care providers are actively working to minimise the use of behaviour modifying drugs in dementia.

In summary

The key issue is to try to gain some understanding of the problem and to match the solution with this understanding. Although caregivers sometimes feel desperate, it is better to try to remain patient and to work methodically through the possible causes and solutions. There are now dementia behavioural advisory services available in most areas of New Zealand.

Chapter 10

Caregiving

Does the road wind uphill all the way?
Yes, to the very end.
Will the day's journey take the whole long day?
From morn to night my friend.
Shall I meet other wayfarers at night?
Those who have gone before.
Then must I knock or call when just in sight?
They will not keep you waiting at the door.
Shall I find comfort, travelsore and weak?
Of labour you shall find the sum.
Will there be beds for me and all who seek?
Yea, beds for all who come.

CHRISTINA ROSSETTI [1]

Care continues throughout life. Caring for a person with dementia begins when that person develops the first signs of dementia, and continues through diagnosis and the various stages as the illness progresses. It does not stop if the person requires residential care. It continues through the terminal phases and into the time of the funeral or other rituals of farewell and remembrance. This whole journey, from the initial signs of dementia to death, might last 20 years or more.

Caring is a process of adaptation, or a journey. The earlier chapters described how dementia progresses and the needs of the person with dementia change. Carers have to be adaptable and flexible, adjusting to changes and involving others as necessary along the way.

> Alzheimer's changes people profoundly and these changes are usually painful to observe. But an important thing to remember is that you will not lose your relationship with the person you are caring for, although you may have to allow your role in this relationship to change.
>
> FRENA GRAY-DAVIDSON [2]

The carer's situation may change independently of the person with dementia: a husband retires and has more time available to care for his wife, a grandchild gets into difficulties leaving a daughter less time for her mother. Older carers suffer from their own health problems and it becomes harder for them to look after their relative.

Who are the carers?

For married people the main caregiver is usually the partner. For those living alone (often women) it is likely to be a daughter or daughter-in-law.

After retirement some men enjoy the chance to develop their 'nurturing' side. They cope admirably caring for a wife with dementia and find the experience fulfilling. However, most of the caring for people with dementia, non-paid and professional, is done by women, most often wives, then daughters and daughters-in-law.

Often the carers are as old as those they care for and may be frail or unwell themselves. In the UK nearly half the carers are over 70 years of age. In the 2001 New Zealand Census, 11 per cent of women over 65 years of age and 10 per cent of men in that age group reported that they looked after someone who was ill or disabled.[3] It is likely a large proportion of those being cared for would have some degree of dementia.

In New Zealand around 70 per cent of people with dementia are cared for in their own homes, usually by one carer.[4] Caregivers might live 24 hours a day in the house of the person with dementia, or they may live in the same area so that they can call in often, or they might live at a distance, keeping in touch and supervising from afar.

Becoming a caregiver

Often people feel they have no choice but to accept the role of caregiver. A spouse may feel obliged to care for a partner. Children who have previously taken parents into their homes may continue to provide care if the parent develops dementia. Traditional cultural patterns may decide who is expected to take on the primary caregiving role — for example, the wife of the oldest son. Usually it is a daughter who takes on the role, but it may depend on which family member lives closest. If one family member says they can't or won't take on the responsibility, another may feel obliged to do so. However, many people willingly take on the role and others just slip into it.

> A very complex, overlapping, sometimes contradictory net of circumstances, relational and gender issues, personal

> inclination and ability to resist obligation decides who becomes the primary caregiver.
>
> ANNE OPIE [5]

Becoming a caregiver can be an emotionally challenging and unsettling experience. It may take years to accept the enormous changes in expectations and lifestyle and the losses associated with this.

Emotional and physical stress

Many studies have attempted to measure the stress that carers are under as they look after someone with dementia. As a group, carers tend to show increased levels of depressive symptoms and anxiety. However, studies also indicate that many people take on caregiving with a sense of vocation; despite feeling tired, worried and frustrated at times, they find that caring is a loving and rewarding task.

In a 1993 UK survey 97 per cent of carers were found to be suffering from some form of emotional difficulty: stress, tiredness, depression or loneliness. Over a third had some form of physical problem, such as back pain, as the result of being a caregiver.[6] Different studies have found that strain is increased if the person with dementia is apathetic (lacking initiative), needs physical care, is incontinent, has disturbed sleep or gets angry easily.

The degree of stress is affected by the nature of the relationship before the cared-for person developed dementia. It may be difficult for someone to accept the role of caring for a person they did not much like even when that person was well. Some spouses feel resentment towards their partners, who by becoming ill have prevented fulfilment of their retirement dreams. Caring out of a sense of duty or guilt will increase the emotional stress on the caregiver. On the other hand, if the relationship has been warm, the family may just accept the situation and get on with the caring with minimal strain.

> *I never thought for a moment that I would not do it. She looked after me with such devotion and love; it was little enough I could do in return to do the same for her.*
>
> A HUSBAND TALKING ABOUT HIS WIFE

> *We took each other for better or worse, so from that point of view I want to care for him the best I can.*
>
> A WIFE SPEAKING OF HER HUSBAND

People are often torn between caring for someone with dementia and other demands on their time. They may be looking after children or grandchildren as well. This can be a difficult balancing act and none of the tasks seem to be done properly.

> *It was very difficult for me and very difficult juggling the demands. There's only one of me and I can only spread myself so thin and that was the trigger that told me I needed some nursing help. He needed twenty-four-hour-a-day attention and there was no way I could give it to him. I could have done it if I didn't have small children, but it was totally out of the question.*
>
> A WOMAN TALKING ABOUT HER STRUGGLE TO LOOK AFTER HER FATHER

COMMON FEELINGS IN CARERS

Embarrassment	*Humour*
Fear and worry	*Hope*
Grief and loss	*Acceptance*
Inadequacy	*Confidence*
Anger	*Understanding*
Resentment and bitterness	*Gratitude*
Guilt	*Forgiveness of self and others*
Depression, hopelessness	*Courage*
Frustration	*Pride in ability to learn and overcome*

Dealing with negative feelings

The emotional state of the person with dementia can communicate itself to those close by, who may also develop similar feelings. For example, if the person with dementia is feeling frightened, their carer may also experience fear. If a carer feels unexpectedly negative, they may be able to step back and recognise that their feelings are a reflection of those of the person with dementia. They then realise they are not 'going crazy' or being irrational, and they can also better understand how the sufferer is feeling. During the course of the illness, most carers learn to not become over involved, yet still remain loving and empathetic.

People have different ways of coping with unpleasant feelings. Here are a few suggestions:

Embarrassment: Accept that what is happening is the result of the illness; explain this to others, and be aware that the embarrassment wears off eventually.

Fear: What are you afraid of? Is it realistic? Can you do anything about it? Talk to other people about how they handled similar situations. If you are a worrier, try distracting yourself with something else when the worries start up.

Grief and loss: What is happening is sad. Have a weep, by yourself or on someone's shoulder. Don't take personally the hurtful things the person with dementia says, especially if such things are out of character.

Inadequacy: No single person is up to the task of caring for a patient throughout the course of dementia. Don't expect the impossible of yourself. Realise you are bound to fail occasionally. Accept help. Congratulate yourself on your ability to cope and learn each day.

Anger: Walk away if you are angry with the person with dementia. Count to 10 before yelling back. Go for a very brisk walk, dig up the garden, yell at something else. Share your angry feelings with a sympathetic person. Write letters to the people you are angry with: friends, the government, the editor, God. You don't have to post them.

Resentment and bitterness: Try to clear the air with the people you feel resentful towards. Forgive them. If it is your situation in general that you resent, how can you change it? People who feel resentful often think they are trapped and powerless. There are always creative choices that can improve life for both parties.

Guilt implies feelings of responsibility. Usually people feel guilty because they can't do what they would like to do, or feel they have failed to live up to their own standards. Check with others how bad you have been. Work out ways to do things better next time. Accept that you are human. Forgive yourself.

Depression and hopelessness: There will be times of despair for everyone. Find someone to talk to or write down your feelings. Try to pinpoint what triggered these feelings and deal with it when you have the strength. Perhaps you have over-reacted because you are too tired, have too much on or aren't taking enough time for yourself.

Frustration: Express your feelings to a friend or write down what is frustrating you. Try to deal with the source of frustration. Recognise that you might be mirroring the feelings of the person with dementia.

Overcome: Write down on a piece of paper everything that is making you feel overwhelmed. Read it, add to it, then burn it and watch it go up in smoke.

Caring for the caregiver

It is easy for carers to focus on the person with dementia and forget about themselves. However, if you don't look after yourself, your health will eventually break down, and you may not be able to continue providing care. Far from being selfish, attending to your own needs is absolutely essential for the sake of the person with dementia.

Accepting help

Caring for someone with dementia is not something people should expect to do on their own. Some find it easy enough to ask for help. Others find it difficult to acknowledge that they are not able to cope. There is no particular reason why one person should expect to be the sole carer for an individual who has a chronic, disabling neurological disease. Men in particular often want to care independently for their wives, but this can mean that they become isolated and lose perspective, perhaps not recognising when their care is inadequate. If the carer refuses help, it is hard for others to know when and whether to offer assistance again. If a sole carer cannot continue, it may be difficult for the person with dementia to accept input from others if no one else has previously been involved with them.

Family and friends

It is a good idea to involve family and friends right from the beginning. Even if carers do not need much help initially, they may need to call on these others at a later date. This is easier to do if potential support people have been kept informed of what is happening. If the main carer explains the situation, friends and family will be more understanding and feel less helpless.

Often other people don't know how to help. Carers can tell them what is valuable. They can suggest specific ways of being involved with the person with dementia, such as visiting while the carer goes out, taking the person for a drive or to watch sports. There may be ways people can support the carer personally; for example, by coming round to chat or making a regular phone call to check on how the carer is.

> *'Our friend G. was great,' says a woman whose husband had dementia. 'He used to pick J. up in the morning in his truck and go out to his landscaping work. To start with, J. could help a bit, but later he just liked to go in the truck and watch what was happening. They did this a couple of times a week for a long time until J. started to wander off. After that G. would come round and sit with him while I went out.'*

People often find it difficult to visit their friends who have dementia. This can leave the main carer feeling isolated and betrayed, and very angry on behalf of their loved one. Some people avoid the person with dementia because they identify with them ('It could be me . . .'), or are just horrified at the change in the person they once knew. Often they stay away because they just don't know what to do or say.

Friends can be helpful in the following ways (see also chapter 13):

- Try to see the situation from the point of view of the carer and the person with dementia. What would it be like for you in that situation? What might you find helpful? Ask what you can do.
- Keep in contact. Make the effort to call in and phone up. Don't expect carers to take the initiative; they have enough on their plate.
- Just asking how things are going helps the carer feel less isolated. Give them a chance to tell you. And listen carefully and try to understand.
- If the person with dementia cannot make conversation, then sit and watch TV with them, listen to music or go for a walk. They will still enjoy your company and interest.
- Take the person with dementia out to places they have previously enjoyed: go for a walk around the golf course, go to the pub or a church. Talk about old times and look at photos. Time spent like this will give the primary caregiver a rest.
- If you and the person with dementia used to go out as part of a group of friends, then continue this. Get an out-of-the-way table in the restaurant if the person with dementia is not great with cutlery. At least keep asking people out, even if they cannot make it. Then they do not feel they have completely disappeared off the face of the earth.
- Offer to do specific chores like the shopping or lawn-mowing. Involve the person with dementia with these tasks if possible.

Whatever happens, don't ignore the person with dementia. It is very hurtful for both the person with dementia and the carer when their friends just drift away.

I rang and said Mum's died, and she said, 'Oh, L., when are you having the service? I would really like to come.' Gosh, if only she'd come when Mum was alive.

And then she said, 'A few months ago I saw this lady in a wheelchair coming towards me as I was walking down the street

> *and I saw it was your mother and I didn't even stop to speak to her.' I thought, God, why didn't she?*
>
> L. TALKING AFTER THE DEATH OF HER MOTHER, WHO HAD VASCULAR DEMENTIA

Alzheimer's New Zealand and other groups

Carer support groups are usually run by the Alzheimer's Society (now called Alzheimer's New Zealand), but sometimes by public hospital teams, rest homes or private hospitals and they can provide both emotional support and practical suggestions. Local Alzheimer's New Zealand branches also run carer education courses, which as well as educating carers give them an opportunity to meet others in a similar situation. Carers can phone their local branch to ask for details. They may want to check whether there is care available for the person with dementia if he or she cannot be left alone while the carer attends a support group. Alzheimer's New Zealand has lots of resources, including field workers to support carers. Some people find the Alzheimer's group vital to their ability to cope.

> *You need to be involved in the Alzheimer's support group. I don't care that people say 'I don't need it'. You do, as far as I'm concerned. I went along and joined. I wasn't going to, because I wasn't a person to go into a circle and tell them about my husband, you know, what is happening in your life, but I tell you what, they were brilliant! There were people there who were ahead of my husband and they could say, 'You know, my wife or husband was similar with the illness'. And they would tell me what they did.*
>
> J. TALKING ABOUT HER EXPERIENCE AS A CARER

Another useful contact is CarersNZ: www.carers.net.nz

Using available services

Carers should make use of all the services that are available, if they are suitable. Some people are grateful if a cleaner can relieve them of household duties, whereas others find cleaning 'therapeutic' and can scrub, sweep and vacuum away their tension. Services that are generally available are listed in chapter 11. It is important that carers make clear what they want, and do not just accept what is on offer. The first point of contact for services is your GP, who can refer you on to a needs assessor.

Looking after physical and mental health

Carers need to take time for themselves on a regular basis. This could be used to participate in their usual hobbies or to meet and relax with friends. It is vitally important to retain a sense of self and not to feel overwhelmed with being 'just a caregiver'. Carers also benefit from holidays or weekend breaks. At these times family or friends might come in to look after the person with dementia, or a more formal arrangement such as carer support respite (short-term care) can be made.

A good diet and regular exercise help carers keep on top of things. Of course, both these are great for the person with dementia too and going for a walk might be an enjoyable way to spend time together.

Getting enough sleep is vital to the health of the carer. If the person with dementia gets up and walks round at night, the carer will probably be too worried to settle. There can be many reasons why a person with dementia has poor sleep (such as a full bladder, pain or the loss of normal sleep patterns as the disease progresses). It is best to ask for help (such as someone to sleep over) early on to avoid becoming exhausted.

If carers develop persistent feelings of anxiety or depression they should see their GP, who can arrange counselling or other psychological help or, if necessary, offer medication. Sometimes the opportunity to talk regularly to a professional whose main focus is on the carer's feelings is enough.

Keeping a sense of humour

Although dementia is a tragic disease, there are often very funny moments and it doesn't hurt to laugh about them. Laughing helps to reduce anger and restores a person to a more rational state when things have got out of proportion. As one caregiver says, 'You do lots of crying, but you have to laugh. If you don't laugh, you'll never get through it.' As laughter reduces the carer's level of tension, it will also relax the person with dementia.

John Bayley, in his book *Iris: A Memoir of Iris Murdoch,* writes:

> Our mode of communication seems like underwater sonar, each bouncing pulsations off the other, and listening for an echo. The baffling moments at which I cannot understand what Iris is saying, or about whom or what — moments that can produce tears or anxieties, though never, thank goodness, the raging frustration typical of many Alzheimer's sufferers — can sometimes be dispelled by embarking on a joky parody of helplessness, and trying to make it mutual. Both of us at a loss for words. [7]

Dealing with professionals

Sometimes people feel intimidated when dealing with the so-called experts in the field of dementia, whether they are specialist doctors, GPs, nurses or volunteers from support organisations. These people are there to help people with dementia and their caregivers. They should recognise that the caregiver is the one who best knows the person with dementia. If the carer has concerns, the professional should take them seriously. Carers should persist in their requests until they feel satisfied with the response they have received. They do not have to take the advice (or the medication) they are given, but they should discuss any reservations they have with the professional making the recommendation. They might then come up with a mutually satisfactory solution.

It often helps to take a friend along to interviews and examinations. A friend can back up the carer and supply information the carer might forget in the heat of the moment. It is a good idea to get the health professional to write down the advice given, to refer to later.

When things go wrong

Physical illness, delirium

People with dementia, like other older people, are prone to physical illness and this may cause a sudden change in behaviour such as increased agitation, drowsiness or poor food or fluid intake. The person with dementia may not be able to explain verbally what is wrong, and there may be no indication of the cause, so an abrupt change in behaviour should be taken to indicate physical illness until proven otherwise. If the cause is a physical illness then it's imperative that treatment is sought promptly. Other causes of behaviour change require less urgent treatment.

The characteristics of delirium, which frequently accompanies physical illness in those with dementia, are listed in chapter 3. Common causes of delirium are infections, reactions to medication, stroke, heart or respiratory problems, or abnormalities of body chemistry and dehydration. Constipation and pain can cause changes in behaviour and need to be treated. Other common physical problems include falls and other accidents, and fractures, particularly hip fractures. If a carer thinks there may be something wrong they should contact their GP as soon as possible. The GP may be able to treat the problem themselves or may refer the patient to a community service that can diagnose and manage the person with dementia in their own environment (with ongoing support and supervision in case things deteriorate).

Going to hospital

It may be necessary to admit a person with dementia to hospital. Going to hospital is difficult enough for people with all their faculties intact. For a person with dementia, and perhaps delirium as well, the sudden change of environment is extremely confusing. Add to that their separation from familiar people, a stream of questions, uncomfortable tests and a rigid hospital regime, and it is surprising that people with dementia ever cope in hospital at all. Pain, noise, sleeplessness, anaesthetics and surgery will also increase their confusion.

Nursing and medical staff tend to focus on the acute problem that has brought the person into hospital and they may not be particularly aware of the ongoing needs of the person with dementia. They may not have had much experience of people with dementia and are likely to be pressed for time on busy medical or surgical wards.

Ideally a family member or other familiar person should stay with the patient during their hospital stay. Some wards make allowance for this, providing a room or a reclining chair for a relative. Often, though, family members are already exhausted from trying to cope with the ill person at home and need a quiet environment to get some sleep. If no one can stay at the hospital, it is helpful to write out any information that could be useful for the hospital staff. This would include such things as:

- What name the person likes to be called
- What help they need generally for their usual activities
- Specific likes and dislikes
- Who to call for further advice
- Particular ways the person communicates
- Other impairments, such as poor vision or hearing.

Tips for how to make a hospital admission easier can be found at www.fightdementia.org.au/understanding-dementia/section-2-caring-for-someone-with-dementia.aspx

If someone is very confused and disruptive, they may need to be treated in a single room. Sometimes a one-to-one nurse (a 'special' nurse) is provided to keep the person safe. Medication may be used to calm the patient, and they may need protective railings to prevent them falling out of bed. Caregivers should be consulted about treatment and should not feel obliged to agree with medical suggestions if they do not think it is in their relative's best interest.

After the acute problem has settled, the patient may be offered rehabilitation in a ward for older people. Family members can also have a say in whether they wish this to happen. Often it is better to get people with dementia back to their familiar environment as soon as possible.

The diagnosis of dementia may be made for the first time while the person is in hospital for something else. It is much better to know about the dementia beforehand to be prepared for the admission.

Loss of caregiver

The sudden death or illness of the caregiver is not uncommon. A person with dementia can be abruptly left on his or her own, dealing not only with day-to-day life but also the stress of bereavement. If one parent has been caring for another, this may be the first time the children recognise how severely disabled the person with dementia is.

It is a good idea to have a contingency plan for such an event. This could involve:

- Regular phone calls or visits to check on the health of the caregiver, as well as the person with dementia.
- Sharing the care with other family members on a regular basis so that there is someone to step in immediately should things go wrong.
- A nominated person who can drop everything at short notice and assist in the immediate period. (This is easier for some people than others.)
- Keeping contact with health services, especially your GP and perhaps the district nurse, social worker or someone else who knows 'the system' and can be called upon for help in an emergency.
- Developing a relationship with a local residential home (maybe somewhere the person has been for respite or day care, so that it is familiar) that could accommodate the person in an emergency.

Emergencies have a nasty habit of occurring in the evenings or on the weekend when the usual professional supports are not available. Some regions have geriatric or psychiatric crisis teams who can arrange short-term carers to come into the home, emergency respite at a rest home or, if necessary, public hospital admission. It is usually best if the person with dementia can remain at home during the crisis so as they don't have the additional stress of having to adjust to new surroundings, people and procedures.

This can be a very difficult time for family members, who may also be bereaved or dealing with life-threatening illness in a loved one. The person with dementia may not understand exactly what is happening, but will sense the changes and be distressed by the absence of the person they normally depend on. This can result in agitation or other disturbed behaviour, which further complicates the situation.

Although families might prefer not to think about the possibility of this type of emergency, it is better to have a plan in place to deal with it than to have to face the trauma unprepared.

In summary

People with dementia can be cared for at home, but this can be stressful for the main caregiver. Carers need to look after themselves and be able to call upon family, friends, Alzheimer's New Zealand and professionals to assist them, both over the long term and in emergencies.

References

[1] Crump, R. W. (ed.), *The Complete Poems of Christina Rossetti*, Louisiana State University Press, Baton Rouge, 1979.

[2] Gray-Davidson, Frena, *Alzheimer's Disease: Everything you need to know*, RGA Publishing Group, London, 1999.

[3] New Zealand Census 2001.

[4] Richards, J., 'Dementia: The privilege of caring', *New Zealand Family Physician*, 28 (1):19–21, 2001.

[5] Opie, Anne, *There's Nobody There: Community care of confused older people*, Oxford University Press, Oxford, 1992.

[6] 'Deprivation and Dementia: A report by the Alzheimer's Disease Society', Alzheimer's Disease Society, London, 1993.

[7] Bayley, John, *Iris: A Memoir of Iris Murdoch,* Duckworth Publications, London, 1998, p. 44.

Chapter 11

Looking after someone at home

Home is where the heart is.

Most people want to continue living in their own homes for as long as possible, despite becoming frail or forgetful. As people age, they may wish to move from a large family home to a smaller house that is easier to heat and maintain. Even in the early stages of dementia, people find it difficult to adapt to new surroundings, so if a move appears inevitable, the sooner it happens the better.

Seventy per cent of people with dementia are cared for at home. The government supports 'Ageing in Place' and is trying to discourage people from going into residential care until absolutely necessary.

The pros and cons of care at home

The benefits

The person with dementia gets what he or she wants

If people with dementia want to keep living in their own homes, we should support this for as long as possible. Then they don't have to face the trauma of leaving their familiar environment: house, garden, belongings, routines, neighbours, clubs, GP and other services. Wanting to stay at home means wanting to remain as independent as possible. For most people, moving into residential care will make them more dependent on others and less able to make their own choices.

Benefits to the caregiver

Husbands and wives, who have shared many years together, usually want to stay together even though one of them has dementia. They can still give each other affection, physical closeness and companionship. Often the carer says, 'She [or he] would have done the same for me, if I'd got dementia'. Husbands and wives feel satisfaction at being able to keep the promise, 'till death do us part'. They may also be honouring an agreement not to put the person into a home.

Many husbands find being a caregiver fulfilling, especially if they have previously not made use of their caring and nurturing side. Looking after a wife who needs them gives meaning to their life which, since retirement, may have lost direction. They fear losing their role and meaning if their beloved spouse goes into residential care.

Daughters (and occasionally sons) may also be in the same position.

Financial benefits

At present, residential care for people over 65 years of age is income- and asset-tested. Putting someone in a rest home means that the person uses up their savings, and if they live alone they may have to sell their house and car to finance care. The longer the person remains at home, the less will have to be paid out for residential care and the more assets can be retained. Older people are often reluctant to spend their savings, as they want to leave something for their family to inherit. A spouse who is much younger than the person with dementia may need to preserve any investments to support them during their retirement.

Keeping people at home benefits the state if care at home is cheaper than residential care. However, good community care can be more expensive than residential care, especially in the later stages of the illness.

The downside of caring for someone at home

For the person with dementia

People with dementia might get poorer care in their own home than in a rest home or private hospital. This could result if there is a difficult relationship between the main caregiver and the person with dementia or if local community services are poorly organised, lack trained staff or are non-existent (as in some distant rural places). The person with dementia may reject help at home, or make it so difficult to provide care that he or she is left alone and at risk of self-neglect or injury. In these cases they might be far better off in a rest home with social contact, good nutrition and medical care. Good residential care can greatly improve a person's mental and physical health. Some people who have struggled for years to live on their own appreciate the security, comfort and company of residential care.

For the caregiver

Caring is a great emotional commitment, requiring time, energy and dedication. Caregivers' health can suffer and they often become socially isolated. They may have to give up leisure activities, looking after grandchildren, travel or other retirement plans. Younger caregivers might have to turn down promotion or give up their job and income.

Financial

Care can be costly if the person doesn't qualify for a Community Services Card. There may be medical costs, payments to housekeepers or carers, private day care and transport to day programmes. Some people resent having to use their savings to pay for care when they had other plans for their future. Others, however, are very willing to pay in order to keep the person at home.

Different types of caring

Living in the same house

Many quite elderly people cope very well looking after their partners who have dementia. Occasionally elderly brothers and sisters live together, supporting each other. As they have known each other for a long time, these elderly caregivers understand the quirks of character of the person with dementia, so tolerate odd behaviour. They often come from a self-sacrificing, independent and non-complaining generation, who accept whatever comes to them as their lot in life. They sometimes find it very difficult to accept help.

Alternatively, an older person may have moved into the home of a child and be living with an extended family. The main carer is then a daughter, son or daughter-in-law, who may or may not have accepted the task willingly. The presence of grandchildren in the home as well as the older person with dementia complicates family relationships because of conflicting demands. Some people come up with creative arrangements to keep people at home.

> *L. arranged for private 24-hour care at home for her parents, who both had dementia. It may not have been much more expensive than residential care for both of them.*
>
> *'. . . the main thing for me was that they were in their own home. They felt comfortable and happy there. I always felt that in a rest home they would be just sitting along the wall.'*

Once dementia is severe and 24-hour care is needed, the main caregiver will need support — both to provide care for the patient and also for regular breaks to recharge his or her batteries. If that can be provided at home then the person with dementia can stay there safely.

Living close by

Sometimes, the caregiver lives nearby and can visit frequently and supervise care. Usually the carer is an adult child who is close enough to call in several times a week. Sometimes the relationship is more distant, for example, a niece taking the main responsibility, or a friend or neighbour. The main carer in this situation can help with certain tasks, such as shopping, bill-paying, cleaning, meal preparation and general supervision. They will be the person called in an emergency. As the neighbours are likely to be the first on the scene if something goes wrong, it is important that they know how to contact the primary caregiver.

While this kind of caring does not involve the 24-hour physical care of the person with dementia, there are different stresses. The main caregiver often has other responsibilities, such as a job or a growing family, and juggling these other needs can prove difficult. Because they are not on the scene all the time, there is always the worry that the person with dementia may be doing something risky in their absence.

> *'In my job,' said M. who watched over her aunt in the same town, 'I drive a lot. So I would just pop in and tell her I was just passing. She'd say, "Well, you won't be staying long then?" And I'd say, "Oh no, no time for a cup of tea", but I was able to check on her.'*

Knowing when to insist on more care or services can be difficult, especially if the person with dementia doesn't see the need for them, cancels them or refuses to pay for them. There may come a time when the main carer just has to tell the person that more paid help is coming in. Fortunately, after a while, the person with dementia may forget his or her objections and the new care becomes part of the routine.

The 'non-resident' caregiver cannot be available for routine care, like toileting, and is not able to provide constant surveillance for people who might put themselves in danger. When dementia is severe and the person needs a lot of physical care or becomes unsafe, this sort of home care is not enough.

Community support

If the person with dementia has no close family, or their family lives at some distance (often, overseas) or is estranged from them, then the main source of support will come from more distant relatives, friends, neighbours, professionals or other community members.

Children who live away from their parents may not have a full understanding of the day-to-day issues affecting someone with dementia. Local people support the person at home and sometimes the children only become aware of problems when there is an emergency. At some point, they may need to decide whether to move closer, to shift the parent to their own community or to consider residential care earlier than they would have if they were living nearby. All of these options are disruptive.

> *'Last week,' says an only son living in Auckland, 'I thought my mother was all right. Then I got a call from the neighbours to say she was in the ambulance on the way to Tauranga Hospital. So I drove down again to see what was happening.'*
>
> *He is waiting for the results of a geriatric assessment before deciding on his next move. He is thinking of bringing her back to live with him in Auckland.*

People living in retirement complexes will still have a relative as the main caregiver although there may be additional support available, such as an emergency call system or the provision of meals.

An intermediate step is to live in a serviced apartment. Often these apartments are associated with aged-care facilities. Care is then shared between the family and staff, who provide a degree of supervision.

Getting help

In most places in New Zealand, there are services to help care for people with dementia at home. To qualify for state-funded home care people have to be assessed by a Needs Assessment Service to make sure they would benefit from the available services. People with dementia can hire private home help if they wish, though it may still be worth talking to the assessment service for recommendations on how to get such help.

Assessment for home care support services

The Needs Assessment and Service Coordination (NASC) services are the people who assess the person with dementia, identify that person's goals and the caregiver's needs and arrange the support service 'package'. Usually, a GP or health care worker refers the patient to NASC. The person with dementia or their family can ask directly for assessment, though most NASC services will want to get medical information from the person's GP.

Older people's NASC services may be run by the DHB, but for younger people the service may be provided by a private organisation contracted by the Ministry of Health. The assessor from NASC visits the person with dementia and their carer at home to find out what the client's needs are. The assessment is usually carried out in the home as this gives a clearer picture of how the person with dementia is able to function in their usual environment. If the assessment is done in hospital (when the person is an inpatient) it will need to be reviewed if the patient returns home. The main caregiver is included in the assessment whenever possible.

An internet-based assessment, interRAI, initially developed for residential care, is also sometimes used in the community. This system is being rolled out throughout New Zealand at the time of writing.

The assessor will discuss the needs assessment with the patient and the family, and make any changes necessary as the result of the discussion. The assessment and its recommendations will be written up and if the person with dementia (or the family) agree with it they will be asked to sign it. A copy of the assessment is left with the patient (or their caregiver). If the patient or family do not agree with the assessment they will be advised on the appeal process.

The assessor may also be the person who discusses services with the person with dementia and caregiver, or there may be a separate service coordinator. The support need is described by a 'scale' or a 'band'. This can range from very low to very high. The bands indicate the approximate amount that may be spent on support services. The service coordinator will explain what the bands mean and decide with the person with dementia and the caregiver what they want. The coordinator will tell them about the services available to meet these needs. Personal care services such as help with showering and dressing are available free for all New Zealanders, but to receive financial assistance with housework, a person needs to have a Community Services Card.

Recently, some NASC services have been doing telephone assessments (usually reassessments). This can have unwanted results if the person with dementia says that services are no longer required! The assessor should always speak to the carer as well.

Choosing which agency to use

Home care services are provided by various organisations that have contracts with the DHB. They are contracted to employ, train, supervise and manage the workers who go into the older person's home to do personal care or other tasks. The agencies fall into three broad categories:

Private agencies (includes individuals offering the service), sometimes operating from a residential care chain.

Non-governmental organisations (NGOs) such as church-based ones (e.g. Presbyterian Support, Enliven) or other charitable bodies.

Marae-based and culture-specific services: There may be such a service in your area, so ask about it if this is what you want.

Some home care agencies are better at caring for people with dementia than others. Some cater for a particular ethnic group. The service coordinator will give you the names of the agencies in the district that provide home care services and ask the person or family to choose which one to use. The coordinator can describe how each agency works and give information about the levels of skill and expertise, but cannot recommend any one service over another. It is often difficult to decide which might be the best agency to use. Carers can get advice from people who are already getting home help, their GP, a hospital social worker or the local branch of Alzheimer's New Zealand. In many areas, however, there is just one agency available, so there is no choice to be made.

Questions you might like to ask about home help and personal care:

- Will it be the same person coming in to help or is there likely to be a series of different people? A team of, say, three consistent people might work but multiple changes of caregiver will be confusing.
- Will they be able to come at the same time each day? It is really important for both the person with dementia and the caregiver that the service is reliable and predictable.
- Are services available seven days a week? Some run only five days a week and this will not be enough if the family is not available to help in the weekend.
- What if the help doesn't turn up? How will you know this if the person who is to be cared for can't remember? Is there a system of recording visits?
- Will the worker be able to handle difficult behaviour? What if the patient refuses to let them in or demands they leave?
- Is there a chance to choose between carers to find someone who might

best suit the patient? For example, a male caregiver may be more suitable for a 'man's man'.

- Are there services available for your particular ethnic or religious group?
- Will there be regular meetings to iron out difficulties? Who do you complain to if you are not happy with the care?

Make sure that the person with dementia's individual needs are met and that you feel reasonably confident that they will be getting the right sort of support.

Community-based care

Home support

Housekeeping: cleaning, laundry, shopping (if no family available).

This can relieve the primary carer of some tasks and may also provide a bit of company for the person with dementia if they live alone, although that is not the main goal. This service is available free to Community Services Card holders.

Personal care

This includes bathing, showering, getting up, dressing, cooking, preparing meals, possibly giving medication (most agencies do not want their staff to be responsible for this but staff will often check to see if medications have been taken).

This is available to all including those who do not have a Community Services Card.

Personal care support helps people function in their basic self-care. For example, someone can visit in the morning, get the person with dementia up and dressed, make their breakfast and supervise the taking of medication. They can come back to prepare lunch and tea and later in the evening put the person to bed. The help should be tailored to the needs of the person with dementia and aim to fit in with other services.

Sitter service

In some areas a 'sitter' comes in to be with a person who cannot be left alone so that the main carer can go out. This can be a regular service or just occasional and can be funded through the carer support scheme (see page 156) or privately. Some people prefer to pay for a sitter out of their own funds and save the carer support days to give themselves a longer break.

Worries about care in the home

Risk of abuse

A person with poor memory is very vulnerable to exploitation and abuse and some people worry that a caregiver coming in may harm their family member. This fear can be heightened if the person with dementia has delusions about the caregiver; for example, that they are stealing the shopping money. There are not many instances of people being exploited or abused and paid caregivers are usually extremely dedicated people who really enjoy looking after older people. (The care-recipient has to sign that the worker has provided the service, e.g., one hour's care. People receiving care are likely to sign whatever they are asked to do — even if not true!) If the family has any concerns about a paid caregiver, they should tell the home care agency. If shopping is part of the job, caregivers should provide receipts for all spending.

Not turning up on time

One of the main complaints seems to be that caregivers don't turn up at the expected time or the time they come isn't convenient; for example, if they come at 10 a.m. to give a shower to someone who gets up at 8 a.m. Apart from asking for a change in time, it is hard to know what else to do, as caregivers have to fit many people into their schedule and may have to deal with unexpected problems.

Many agencies leave a book at the house of the person with dementia so that the caregivers can record the visit and note what has been done. This allows relatives to reassure themselves that what was planned has actually happened.

Personality clashes

Occasionally there is a personality clash between the carer and the person being cared for. This might mean that the carer has to be replaced. Some people with dementia make it very difficult for people trying to help, but often an experienced worker will be able to smooth the way.

If the patient is physically violent or demands that the caregiver leave, there is not a lot that care agencies can offer. The home care worker is an employee of the agency and expects the employer to provide a safe workplace. No one can be expected to place themselves at risk of persistent verbal abuse or in physical danger. Severe incontinence can also be difficult to manage at home over the long term.

Requests for change

At the time the care is set up, the organiser should give the family (or other involved people) the name of the person to contact if they are not satisfied or if they require any changes. The family will need to contact the agency if care is no longer required (e.g. if the person goes into hospital). They should also set up regular meetings to review the situation. The original NASC service coordinator will be available to help if there are concerns.

Carer support

People who care for someone at home may be allocated a certain number of days each year of carer support. This means that someone else will look after the person with dementia for a specified amount of time. This is government recognition that looking after someone long term is exhausting and the carer needs regular breaks. People who live with someone with dementia or provide at least four hours' care per day qualify for carer support (usually up to 28 days per year). NASC services can allocate more if necessary.

The days can be used however the caregiver chooses. For example, if the main caregiver wanted a whole month off on holiday, the person with dementia could stay for four weeks in a rest home. On the other hand, if the carer wanted an afternoon off every week to go shopping, then a worker could come in for half a day per week to sit with the person with dementia or the person could go to a day programme (day care).

Day care

Day care is when the person with dementia goes out during the day on a regular basis (to a day care centre, rest home or private hospital) to join a group of older people participating in various activities run by trained staff. The usual hours are 10 a.m. till 2 or 3 p.m. and a meal is provided at lunchtime. Theoretically, a person could attend every weekday, but for most people more than one or two days a week is too tiring. Some areas have (or are developing) seven-day-a-week programmes, so that people with dementia can attend at the weekend.

The goal of day care is to offer a stimulating activity programme and to allow social contact between older people who might otherwise be isolated at home. It also relieves carers for a few hours and provides additional supervision of people living on their own who might not be able to recognise a problem they have or ask for help.

It can be difficult to persuade someone with dementia to go to day care. It is a strange and, at least initially, frightening environment. The main caregiver can go with the person for the first few times, gradually leaving them for longer and longer periods. As well as settling the person with dementia, this reassures the caregiver that their family member is in good hands. Once they get used to it, many people enjoy the outing. Some people (especially older men) see it as going to 'work' or the club.

Day care is not always successful. Some carers say that it is hardly worth the effort given the stress of getting the person there and dealing with their agitation when they get home. For others, despite the organisation involved, it is worthwhile, even essential.

> *J. says, 'I used to have it down to a fine art. I would get myself up in the morning, get myself ready, have my breakfast, then I'd get him up. I would bath him or shower him and I would give him his breakfast — help him with his breakfast. He would have a piece of toast here, but when he went down to W. Day Care they would give him his porridge and then he would have his lunch down there and I would bring him home. I could have left him there seven days a week until 9.00 at night, but I wouldn't . . .'*

Types of day care

Day care may be general, that is, groups that are run for older people who do not necessarily have dementia. These are suitable for people with mild to moderate dementia, who can manage social situations reasonably well. Carer support may be used towards the cost of general day care; otherwise, there is no subsidy.

Dementia day care is set up especially for people with dementia and other people are not accepted. The programmes are designed with dementia sufferers in mind. The day care centre is often associated with a residential dementia unit, so that suitable staff and equipment are available.

If the person is assessed by a NASC team as needing dementia day care then it is usually free, though sometimes there is a small charge for transport. This may vary in different DHB areas.

Respite care

This is when the person with dementia goes to stay in a residential facility to give the caregiver a break. Carer Support pays for 28 days — or more if this is assessed as necessary. A carer who wants more may pay privately. There is usually a significant 'top up' charge as the government does not cover the full cost of residential care in this situation. This means that less well-off people often cannot afford respite care.

Intermittent care

In addition to carer support, some (but not all) District Health Boards pay for intermittent care, which gives the carer a more frequent regular break. The person with dementia spends six to 10 weeks at home with their usual caregiver and then one or two weeks in a rest home or private hospital. This means that every two or three months (more or less, as arranged with the intermittent care service) the caregiver can get time off. While in residential care, the person with dementia gets the benefit of the activities and can be reviewed by the nurses, who get to know them over time. Because these beds are rostered out to other families using the service, the time limits are strict, although occasionally it may be possible to use an intermittent care bed in an emergency. Regular intermittent care (or respite) helps the person with dementia to become familiar with a rest home. If they subsequently need to go there permanently, then it is not such a shock.

Concerns about respite care

It can be very difficult to decide to put someone in respite or intermittent care and caregivers often wait until they are absolutely exhausted before they do so. People may feel conflicting emotions about using respite care:

- Worries that staff won't be able to manage the person with dementia the way the primary carer can; concern about lack of individualised care and the potential failure of formal caregivers to take notice of the main carer's recommendations.
- Feelings that people with dementia will see themselves as being betrayed or prepared for permanent residential care.
- Expectation of deterioration in the person's skills, especially if staff at the home or hospital are rushed and do not allow the person time to follow their usual routine or if there are no proper day programmes or the person with dementia gets much more confused in a different environment.
- Guilt about taking time out and accepting this sort of help.
- Loneliness and lack of structure to the carer's day.
- Relief to have some time to oneself, enjoyment of catching up on their own life and resentment about having to take up the burden of caring again.

I could have so many days' respite, but I wouldn't use it. If we went away for the weekend, I would take him. It was only the last year, when I was run ragged, but I used to feel so guilty if I put him there and would be crying all the time. I had to do it for me . . .

If the carer has concerns about the care of the person with dementia, talking to the people providing the care should help. Friends, family, your GP or counsellors can help you cope with feelings of guilt. *Remember, caregivers need a break from time to time so that they can carry on caring.*

Night and evening care

Funding via a carer support programme can be used to employ someone to stay overnight to allow the main caregiver to get some sleep. Some people also pay for this privately through one of the private nursing agencies. Night care in a rest home may be available in some places to cater for people who stay awake at night and disrupt the caregiver's sleep.

If the person with dementia goes to a rest home in the early evening, this allows the main caregiver to go out for recreation or entertainment.

For information on available support services go to www.health.govt.nz/publication/needs-assessment-and-support-services-older-people-what-you-need-know

District Health Board (public) services

Day programmes (Day Hospital or Day Ward)

These are usually time-limited programmes to medically assess (and if possible rehabilitate) the person with dementia and to set up longer-term support via other services. They are run by the older person's services at most hospitals. Some mental health services for older people also run day programmes. They are free and transport is often provided.

Dementia advisory services

Recently the government has funded dementia advisory services for each of four regions (Northern, Midlands, Central and South). The goal of these services is to provide information and support for dementia care. Contact details are in the appendix.

Nursing

District nurses (from the hospitals or other organisations, such as Nurse Maude in Christchurch) can assess and provide expert care in such areas as dressing wounds, managing diabetes, and medication education.

Psychiatric district nurses are involved in the assessment phase and can help out if the person has behavioural or psychological difficulties. They may become involved in a crisis situation, especially if the Mental Health Act (see chapter 17) has to be enforced.

Incontinence advice

Some hospitals or other organisations have specific continence nurses (or the service may be provided by district nurses) who can advise on bladder and bowel management and, if necessary, supply products to manage incontinence (wetting or messing). These products include pads, adult incontinence pants (often just for night-time use) and waterproof underblankets. Continence advisors work from the hospital (usually as part of the older people's services). Your general practitioner can make a referral.

House alterations

An occupational therapist (OT) can assess the safety of the home situation and make recommendations. These might be simple, such as the removal of rugs to prevent tripping, or installing a smoke alarm. Or there might be more major changes to make, such as replacement of the bath with a shower, putting in a ramp, handrails, etc. There is usually funding available to pay for this, and the OT can help with finding a builder. Generally OTs work from the hospital, though there are a few private ones around. Your GP or a NASC service assessor should be able to refer you or arrange an OT visit.

Other health professionals

Physiotherapists, speech therapists, dietitians, diversional therapists and social workers also provide assistance in the community (see chapter 7).

Non-governmental organisations

Field workers, carers' support groups and short courses

Alzheimer's New Zealand branches, Stroke Foundation, other non-governmental organisations and public hospitals run support groups so that relatives of people with dementia can share their experiences and develop expertise. Carer education courses help people to understand about dementia and how to deal with the associated challenges. Many people find these groups an absolute lifeline, as they reduce the isolation that affects so many caregivers. Being with a group of people who understand and accept what is happening can be very affirming and helps to improve confidence. To find a group, contact your local branch of Alzheimer's New Zealand (0800 004 001).

Community groups

These include care and craft groups, church groups, etc. For the person with dementia, a regular outing is stimulating, and it can provide a break for the caregiver. However, most groups are run by volunteers and they may find it difficult to tolerate disruptive behaviour such as calling out or walking away. On the other hand, people often bend over backwards to accommodate a person well known to them, even if he or she just drinks tea while watching other people join in the activities.

> *The members of a bingo group helped one of their long-standing members cover her numbers after she developed dementia. When she did not really understand the game, but still came along, they gave her the occasional prize anyway. She really enjoyed going and always had her hat and coat on, ready to leave, hours before the bingo was due to start.*

Visitors

Some church or voluntary agencies provide visitors to lonely older people. They may not always be experienced in dealing with people with dementia.

Caring callers

St John's Ambulance Service has volunteers who regularly phone people who are on their own. They provide company, monitoring and sometimes can remind people to take their medication.

Volunteers

These may be available through Age Concern or Alzheimer's New Zealand.

Other care systems

Medic Alert bracelets

It can be useful for the person with dementia (particularly if they sometimes get lost) to have a bracelet or pendant to identify that they have dementia and to supply carer contact details. A man can also have details in his coat pocket, or for a woman, in her handbag.

Technology

There are many devices available to make care easier and safer. These include:

- prompts and reminders — from simple whiteboards to electronic messages when time to take medicine
- sensory, e.g., electronic pets
- communication aids, e.g., picture cards when verbal language is lost
- safety systems such as electronic monitors to track people who have left home. WandaTrak is often used in New Zealand
- monitoring systems, e.g., fall detectors
- everyday living such as irons that turn themselves off.

Western Australia Alzheimer's has an interesting website, www.fightdementia.org.au/western-australia/assistive-technology---product-information-sheets.aspx. Much of this technology is available in New Zealand or can be ordered from overseas.

Fire brigade

Fire safety officers can advise on fire safety in the house and will install fire alarms (information on www.fire.org.nz).

General practitioner and nurse

The GP will be the main medical person advising on dementia care and keeping an eye on the health of the caregiver. The practice nurse may be a useful support person. She can visit and answer queries, though she may not have had much training in dementia. Some GP practices have a nurse specifically trained in the care of older people available to visit homes and organise care. There are now many geriatric nurse practitioners who are a great source of information and support and are able to prescribe a limited number of drugs for older people.

Financial

A full-time caregiver, who is not a superannuitant, such as an adult child, may be entitled to the Domestic Purposes Benefit. Work and Income (WINZ) can let people know whether they are eligible. WINZ may also pay for additional costs of care, such as doctor's visits, transport or medication via a supplementary allowance.

Advocacy

Alzheimer's New Zealand, Age Concern or the Health and Disability Commissioner may be able to help if you think you are not getting a fair deal from any service provider.

When care at home is too difficult

There is likely to come a time when the disadvantages of caring for a person at home outweigh the benefits and you have to start thinking about residential care. Any or all of the following factors may need to be taken into account:

The care may become too demanding: Frequent incontinence, poor sleep patterns, behaviour disturbances and loss of mobility make it very difficult to look after someone at home.

The main carer's health may deteriorate because of stress: Physical or mental illness may be caused or made worse by the constant worry and exhaustion associated with caring for someone as the dementia progresses.

The person living alone is at risk: People on their own may be in physical danger from falls, fires or abuse from other people. They may neglect themselves and not eat, keep warm or take vital medical treatments. They may refuse to allow community services into the home.

The main carer may not have enough support: Sometimes the loss of an important support person (such as a sister dying or a daughter moving away) is the trigger to consider placement for the person with dementia.

Other needs, e.g. from children or partner, may become more demanding: A daughter may need to decide between caring for a parent with dementia and an ill husband. Children may grow to an age where they need more of their mother's time and energy and she has less available for her own mother.

Insufficient support services in the community: Many communities can provide home visits up to four times a day, but more than that is not usually feasible.

The care isn't good enough: The person has repeated hospital admissions with symptoms of self-neglect or abuse.

> *Mrs A. had help coming in four times a day for many months, but one night, the neighbours found her at the letterbox looking for her mail. On a second occasion, the morning caregiver found her on the floor between her bed and the wall, cold, confused and unable to get up. After a period in hospital everyone decided that it was too risky to try to send her home again.*

The decision is not an easy one and often not helped by well-meaning people blithely advising the main carer to 'put him into a home . . .' without considering the carer's feelings about giving up the role.

These feelings might be:

- grief about losing the physical and emotional presence of a loved one, especially a spouse who has lived with their partner for decades
- guilt about 'letting their family member down'
- fear that the care that they receive will not be good enough and not take individual needs into account
- fear that they will now be excluded from involvement in decisions about the person with dementia
- resentment or anger about the inadequacy of support from family or community services
- doubts about what to do with all the time now available to them.

All these feelings may be mixed with fatigue, a sense of relief at having made a decision and hopefulness about having more time to oneself. Sharing these feelings with a sympathetic friend or relative, an Alzheimer's New Zealand field worker, a counsellor, social worker or your GP can also help.

In summary

Care at home can be challenging but rewarding. Despite the services now available, it is often not possible to keep someone at home through the entire course of their illness. In the next chapter I discuss how to go about making the decision and organising admission into residential care.

Chapter 12

Choosing residential care

Over half of people in residential care had difficulty remembering. This is an indication of the high prevalence of dementia amongst this population group. (This compares with about 7% of people living in standard households.)

MINISTRY OF HEALTH [1]

Despite the negative stereotypes of rest homes and private hospitals, many older people find living in residential care enjoyable. For some it is a relief not to have to worry about running their own home and doing chores that had become enormously difficult. They no longer feel isolated and vulnerable and are pleased to be 'less of a burden' to their children. Although most people do not want to go into residential care it can be a positive move, which improves the quality of life for a person with dementia.

When residential care becomes necessary, people with severe dementia may no longer be able to understand why they need care. Their family, with the social worker, hospital doctor and general practitioner, must make the decision for them.

However, many people can still have some input into the decision. If they are at an earlier stage of Alzheimer's disease (perhaps with physical illness complicating the picture) or have vascular dementia, they might still be able to discuss aspects of the proposed change. They may be able to tell family what they want in a rest home and go on visits to look around premises.

Not everyone will agree that their relative needs to move. Children sometimes strongly object to their parent going into residential care. They may feel that it is the family's responsibility to care for their own, or may have had bad experiences in the past with the care given to other relatives. Sometimes they deny that the person is so disabled that he or she needs 24-hour professional care. Unresolved long-standing family conflicts can be at the base of the disagreement, as in the following case:

Mrs R. looked after her husband, who had severe dementia and arthritis. Despite her daughters' support and maximum home help, she decided to place Mr R. in residential care. She chose a suitable place for him close to where they lived.

At this point Mr R.'s son, G., appeared on the scene, insisting that Mrs R. continue to care for his father. If she did not, G. said he would take his father to his own home (some distance away) to look after him.

It emerged that Mrs R. was Mr R.'s second wife and that the family had been bitterly divided when he remarried. G. had never accepted his stepmother. Mrs R. had not informed him of his father's potential move, perhaps hoping to avoid conflict. Eventually, after much argument, the family accepted Mrs R.'s decision.

The cost of care and subsequent loss of inheritance may be an unspoken motive for avoiding residential care.

The best method of dealing with arguments is to sit down as a family and let everyone have their say. Family members need to know about the person's condition and why he or she might need full-time care. It takes a lot of skill and determination to focus on the issue at hand (where the person with dementia should live) and not to drag in old business and resentments. Often a social worker, hospital doctor or GP can help by overseeing a formal family meeting.

Family meetings can come up with productive solutions or compromises. For example, family members may suddenly realise what a huge strain the main caregiver is under. They can then offer support (such as having the person with dementia to stay) so that the caregiver can cope for longer. Or everyone may agree to a trial at a suitable rest home, to be reviewed after a set time. The people who object to the person with dementia going into care can be asked to look after him or her for a period. Often a weekend in the caregiving role is enough to convince the doubters that residential care is for the best.

Admission to long-term residential care is tightly controlled in New Zealand to avoid people moving into care unnecessarily. Even people who expect to be paying for care privately need an assessment before placement is approved. (This is because they might run out of money and ask for a government subsidy. The government does not want to pay for people who do not need care.)

In most areas, the same Needs Assessment and Service Coordination (NASC) team that arranges support at home will also assess suitability for residential care. The assessor fills in a form and decides on the person's level of need, including whether they require specific dementia care. The person with dementia will also be seen by a geriatrician or psychiatrist to check for medical or psychiatric conditions that could be treated, allowing them to be more independent and to stay at home longer. Placement in a dementia-specific facility must be approved by a psychogeriatrician (a psychiatrist who works with older people).

Types of residential care

Private hospitals

Hospitals provide 24-hour-a-day registered nursing staff to look after people who are very ill or disabled and require a high level of care. Older people needing hospital care are likely to be very frail, immobile or have difficult-to-manage medical conditions. Often they will require two people to move them and they are unable to attend to their own self-care. They need regular monitoring to ensure they remain comfortable and have the best possible quality of life.

Hospitals providing this sort of care are referred to as private hospitals to distinguish them from public hospitals, which rarely provide long-term care. Some private hospitals are run by not-for-profit organisations such as churches or other charitable trusts, but most are commercial ventures.

Rest homes

Rest home residents are more robust. They can attend to much of their own care, but require more supervision and support than can be provided in their own homes. Generally they are mobile enough to need, at most, only one assistant to get around. Many people with moderately severe dementia manage in ordinary rest homes if they are reasonably settled and the staff have some training in dementia care.

Rest homes provide 24-hour staffing, but there is not always a registered nurse on site. A nurse will visit for a specified number of hours per week and be able to be contacted in an emergency. Rest homes are run by private businesses or non-profit organisations.

Specialist dementia care

People with dementia who exhibit behaviours that require specialist skills (such as wandering or hitting out) will be better in a dementia care facility. These facilities are specially designed rest homes or private hospitals whose staff are trained in dementia care.

Dementia-specific rest homes

Rest homes for people with dementia cater for mobile people with dementia. Staff are trained to help the residents retain their skills, to manage difficult behaviour and to organise suitable activities. Ideally (but not always) the buildings are designed with safe indoor and outdoor walking areas and places for people to go for quiet time. The layout should make it easy for people to be viewed unobtrusively by staff. Often dementia-specific units are part of a rest home or private hospital complex. They may also offer day-patient services.

Hospitals for people with dementia (psychogeriatric hospitals)

People who have more complex needs such as increasing frailty, plus difficult behaviour patterns (or very challenging behaviour), are best in a specially designed hospital. The workforce in such hospitals is trained in dementia management as well as being able to attend to physical problems and end-of-life care. These facilities require intensive input and high staffing numbers. They are few and far between.

Monitoring standards in residential care

The MOH contributes to the cost of residential care and in return the residential facilities contract to meet certain standards. These relate to all aspects of residential care: fire safety, food quality, complaints procedures, staff numbers, training and so on. In dementia-specific environments the caregivers must be educated about dementia. The MOH audits these homes and hospitals to ensure standards are maintained. In 2003, the MOH handed the management of these contracts to the District Health Boards, which have taken on the monitoring role.

Confused?

The whole business of assessment and placement changes frequently.

At the present time, 'interRAI' is the assessment tool that is being (or about to be) used in most areas. This international computer-based system is being rolled out to all District Health Boards and determines what level of support an individual needs.

The types of residential care available are:

- Rest homes
- Dementia-specific units or rest homes
- Hospitals
- Psychogeriatric hospitals.

The assessor will tell the family which is the most suitable place for the person with dementia. For example, a frail, placid person with very advanced dementia could be managed in an ordinary private hospital, but someone equally frail who called out a lot and resisted being cared for would need specialist psychogeriatric care.

Choosing a place

The care coordinator (usually the same person as the assessor) supplies the names of places that would be suitable for the person with dementia. The coordinator is not supposed to recommend one place over another. The family has to decide on the best place, and may find the following suggestions helpful.

Going somewhere you know

If the person with dementia has been attending day care at a rest home, the family may have already discussed the possibility of long-term care. In this situation, the surroundings may be familiar and the staff will know about the person with dementia so that the transition is a little easier.

Talking to others

Families who already have someone in care will be able to say what was important to them, how they chose a place and whether they have been satisfied with the care given. The local branch of Alzheimer's New Zealand can help, as can the GP or hospital service.

The Residential Care Line (run by the Auckland District Health Board) gives advice: www.adhb.govt.nz/rcline. Eldernet lists rest homes and private hospitals: www.eldernet.co.nz.

Research

The facilities shown to be the best at maintaining thinking abilities, language, social and self-care skills, as well as reducing agitation and improving mood in people with dementia, have the following features:

- Residents who have been fully assessed and diagnosed
- Staff who are specialised in dementia care and have ongoing education
- An absence of physical restraints or excessive sedating medication
- Care routines that are flexible, and individual care plans for each resident
- An environment that is designed or adapted to suit people with dementia.

Visiting rest homes or private hospitals

To look at a rest home or private hospital either make an appointment to meet the manager or visit unannounced. Go along at different times of the day so that you get a broad picture. (All options should be acceptable to the home or hospital.) Take another person along with you — they may see things that you don't, and it is useful to be able to discuss the visits with them later.

Talking to the manager

Things to ask about when talking to the manager are:

The admission agreement: This shows which items and services are *not* part of standard care and the additional charges for them. Take it home to study and compare it with other rest homes' admission agreements. If you have particular requirements (or objections to the agreement), these can be discussed with the manager.

Staffing: What is the ratio of care staff to residents on each shift? Are they trained in dementia care? Will they be able to manage this person's particular behaviour? What is the policy on restraint? Is there a registered nurse, trained in dementia, in charge of the unit in the day time? At other times, is there a registered nurse on site or on call?

Care plan: Each resident should have a plan to help them maintain skills and give them the best possible quality of life. The family and the resident should help to develop the care plan. How often will the plan be reviewed? What if the family wants to make changes? Will the family be involved in review meetings? Ask to have a look at a sample care plan.

Management questions: Does the manager seem approachable, in case problems come up? What is the overall philosophy, e.g., The Eden Alternative is an approach to reduce loneliness, helplessness and boredom (www.edenalt.org). Are there other levels of care on the same site? (The person with dementia might need to move from the rest home to hospital care or to specific dementia care. It is often easier if the person stays on the same site.)

Activities: What meaningful activities are available? Is someone employed to organise activities for people with dementia? How many hours per week? Are there activities in the late afternoon when people with dementia get restless? What outings are there and how does the person get to go? (People with moderate–severe dementia won't be able to sign themselves up to go for outings.) How often will the person be able to go on an outing? Are there any particular programmes aimed at people with dementia, e.g., Spark of Life (www.dementiacareaustralia.com).

Meals: Ask residents and families about the food. Are there dietary options, e.g., vegetarian food or finger food? If someone is disturbed at mealtimes, is there a quiet place to eat? Are there enough staff to assist with eating, e.g., cutting up food and helping people feed themselves? What times are meals? Will they provide snacks at other times? (This is especially important for people who walk a lot.)

Other services: Enquire about things that are important to the potential resident. Can the person have a shower every day? Can residents keep their own GP or do they have to go to a doctor employed by the facility? Will their own GP be able to visit? For an extra weekly or lump sum payment, better accommodation, e.g., larger room, ensuite, sitting area, may be available. These are known as 'premium rooms'.

Environment: Can (or must) residents bring in their own furniture and other belongings? What about pets? (Who looks after them?) Is a phone available? Can the person visit the hairdresser regularly?

Looking around

Staff: Does the staff member showing you around respect people's rooms as their private space and not enter without knocking or requesting permission? How do the caregivers interact with the residents? Are they involved with them or away doing other things?

Residents: Are the residents alert and active? Are they involved in enjoyable activities?

Bedrooms: Would the available room meet the person's own preferences, e.g., for sunshine, a view, quietness or busyness? If the person is in a private hospital, the rooms are sometimes shared to make nursing easier. In this case, will the person have sufficient privacy?

Bathroom: Most people prefer an en suite bathroom, and this may make it easier for someone with dementia to find the toilet facilities. However, if the dementia is severe the ensuite may be a nuisance as people sometimes dismantle taps, overflow the basin or block the toilet.

Common areas: Does it feel homely? Is it in tune with the person's own home and tastes? Relatives are often impressed by smart places with modern décor, but the person with dementia might prefer something from an earlier era. Are the seats arranged so that people can interact with each other? Is there space for people to walk around easily without interfering with others? Does the dining room seem a pleasant and calm environment (mealtimes are often very stressful for people with dementia).

Quiet areas: Are there smaller areas where someone could go to talk to visitors or get away from others?

Grounds: Is there a nice garden with sheltered seating? Are there places to wander or pace? Is it safely fenced, but in a way that doesn't feel shut in?

Other: Is there an indoor smoking area (if necessary). Is the temperature right? Older people are not so active and need warmer surroundings than younger people.

What if there's no vacancy?

After all the effort of choosing, there may be no vacancy at the home the family has finally decided upon. If the situation is urgent, the patient will have to go to the second-best option until a place becomes available in the preferred home. It is best to tell the manager of the second-choice home that the person is on the waiting list for another home and will be transferred out in due course. It is possible that when a vacancy finally becomes available the person with dementia will be settled and happy in their current place, and the family will decide against another move.

Once people are in residential care, it does not mean they have to stay there. It is quite possible that they could improve and want to try living at home again. The family's circumstances could change and make it possible for the person with dementia to live with them. Perhaps there will be an opportunity to provide paid care at home. People can leave residential care. They don't have to stay there permanently.

Costs

The government contributes to the cost of residential care for certain people living in rest homes or private hospitals. Not everyone is eligible for a *residential care subsidy*. Eligibility is determined by income- and asset-testing: how much people earn and how much they own.

Asset-testing for residential care was being gradually phased out, however the government has stopped this process and the maximum assets to be retained will remain at the 2012 level for the meantime.

Work and Income New Zealand (WINZ) carries out the financial means assessment of the potential resident. The person who is going into care or their agent (such as a family member) fills in forms and provides proof of how much income, property, cash and other financial assets they have.

To be eligible for the residential care subsidy the person needs:

- To be over 65 (though there are some exceptions)
- To have been assessed as needing permanent residential care
- If single or widowed, to have assets, including house and car, worth less than $213,000.
- If married with both partners in residential care, to have assets, including house and car, worth less than $213,000
- If only one of a couple is in residential care, their spouse can keep the house and the car and get a subsidy if they have less than $116,000 in other combined assets (or can opt for the $213,000 level — whichever suits best).

People aged 50–64 are not asset-tested. However, if they do *not* have dependent children, they are income-tested.

What are assets?

- Cash or savings
- Investments, shares or stocks
- Loans made to other people, including family trusts
- House and car if the person lives alone.

Exceptions (i.e. these assets don't count):

- House, chattels and car if partner or dependent child still lives at home
- Personal belongings such as clothing and jewellery
- Pre-paid funeral expenses of up to $10,000 each for the person and their partner.

It is possible to get an interest-free loan from WINZ towards residential care if the person does not want to sell their house or if it is difficult to do so. When the house is sold the loan is repaid.

If the person with dementia or the spouse has an income, this income will have to be paid towards the residential care of the person with dementia. Income includes:

- New Zealand Superannuation, any pension or income support payment
- Overseas government pensions
- Contributions from relatives

- Accident insurance payments
- Earnings from investments or business
- Income from a family trust
- Dividends from stock or bonds.

Exceptions:

- WINZ counts only 50 per cent of private superannuation schemes and annuities
- War Disablement Pension.

For a clear description of financial assistance, see www.workandincome.govt.nz/documents/residential-care-subsidy.pdf

When does the government pay?

If the person meets the criteria for the full subsidy (i.e. few assets and little income, as above) the government pays the total cost of care. Even if a person has too much in the way of income or assets to qualify for the subsidy, there is a maximum they pay towards private hospital, rest home or dementia care (in 2012 this figure was $812–$892 according to district). The DHB will pay a top-up subsidy to cover the higher costs of the sort of care that has been recommended. Check with the NASC assessor for the most current 'maximum contribution'.

When someone has used up their assets, they (or their family) can apply for the full subsidy.

What does a subsidy pay for?

People entitled to a full subsidy receive care including the following services without additional cost. (This does not apply to people paying privately, who may receive different services for their fees.)

- Accommodation
- Meals
- Cleaning
- Laundry
- Emergency doctor's visits plus monthly or three-monthly GP visits as necessary
- Most medications and any required packaging
- All dressings and supplies used in treatments
- Incontinence aids
- Equipment and mobility aids (for communal use)
- Activities

- Physiotherapy, speech therapy, dietician, podiatry, if prescribed by a doctor
- Temporary absences: subsidy will be paid for up to six weeks if the person is away, e.g., with family for a holiday, or three weeks if admitted to a public hospital
- Transport for health reasons, e.g., to a dental or outpatient clinic appointment, and someone to accompany the person if there are no family members available
- Personal allowance ($42.38 per week in 2012) and clothing allowance ($265.81 per year in 2012). This is adjusted according to the consumer price index (CPI).

Work and Income New Zealand (phone 0800 999 727, fax 0800 999 199) can give further, up-to-date advice.

What do private payers get?

If the person is paying privately for care, it is important to find out exactly what the fee covers, as it will not be the same as that provided to subsidised residents. (However, the list above gives some idea of the sorts of things to ask about.) The rest home agreement should detail what the basic fee covers and which items incur additional charges. Commonly these are medications, doctor's fees, incontinence aids and en suite facilities. Note, there has been a recent move by some care providers to offer 'premium rooms' which have additional space or facilities for an extra cost ($20–$30 a day or more).

For further information you can access Ministry of Health (2010), *Long term residential care for older people: what you need to know*, on www.moh.govt.nz, or call the information line (0800 737 777).

Telling the person with dementia

If people with dementia and their families have previously talked about the possibility of residential care, the decision to go ahead with this might not come as a shock. The person with dementia can look at a few suitable facilities, spend some time there during the day, get to know the staff and other residents and decide which is the best place for them.

However, if there has been a sudden collapse of care at home or an abrupt deterioration in the person's health, the decision may have to be made quickly. Even then, it is most respectful to tell the person with dementia that everyone considers that safe care at home is no longer possible. Whether or not the person agrees, at least there is a chance to be open with them, to show them suitable places and take their personal preferences into account. Sometimes this openness complicates things: the person might refuse to consider care and say they don't like anywhere they are shown. Families then have to try other approaches.

If the person is in hospital when the decision is made, they might like to go home to sort out their things and farewell the house before moving into residential care. This can sometimes be tricky! People may be reluctant to leave again and have even been known to barricade themselves in.

What if the person won't go?

Unfortunately, people may lose insight into their disabilities and do not believe that they cannot care for themselves without help . . . 'Don't worry about me, I can look after myself,' they say, when it is clearly not the case. Some determinedly cling on to the wish to remain 'independent' in their own home (something we usually admire).

Below are a number of approaches that can be used to get people to go into care. They begin with the persuasive and end with the legally coercive. People using these approaches need to be convinced that:

- the person's quality of life will be better in residential care
- all relevant objections from the person have been addressed or
- he or she is so impaired in decision-making capacity that someone else should make the decision in their best interest.

This is a very difficult situation: one in which there seems to be only bad outcomes and the family has to pick the least negative.

The concerted family effort: Having the whole family come together to state that the person needs more care than can be provided at home may persuade the person to try residential care. If everyone is of the same mind, the person with dementia might agree to a trial (at least) in a rest home or hospital.

Getting someone that the person with dementia respects to make the case: Often an older person will listen to someone perceived to be 'in authority'. This person could be their GP, a hospital specialist, a priest or minister, a successful son or daughter returning from overseas or their older brother. The people who know the person with dementia will be able to decide who might be the best person to ask. It can go against the grain to bring in these so-called experts when the actual expert, the main caregiver, is treated with disdain, but this approach often works.

Going in for a trial period or for respite: The hope is that the person will have a brief spell in care, like it and be happy to stay. Someone with dementia will need at least three to four weeks to get used to a new situation, so the minimum trial period should be a month. If the person settles down and adapts (as is often the case) then everyone can breathe a sigh of relief.

Going via the hospital: Often older people who resist care for dementia or any form of mental illness will accept a hospital admission for a physical health problem. If someone has back pain, suffers from falls, has difficulty walking or other physical problems, they could be admitted to an older people's ward for assessment, treatment and rehabilitation (ATR). One of the advantages of hospital admission is that a full assessment can be done, and it will become clear either that there is no way that the person can continue at home or that things can be improved and the person can last at home a bit longer. Once treatment is completed, the geriatric team can inform both the patient and the family of the need for residential care and can help arrange suitable placement. It is easier to move people who are already out of their familiar surroundings to a new place than to take them directly from home.

> *M.'s aunt, Miss P., had always been stubborn and independent. As her dementia progressed, she had more and more difficulty with self-care, but would not accept help from anyone but M. (who lived across town). M. became increasingly concerned about her aunt's safety, but Miss P. adamantly refused to consider rest home care.*
>
> *When Miss P. broke a bone in her foot, she was in considerable pain, but did not remember to take her painkilling medication. Eventually, she agreed to go into the local ATR ward where they could treat her foot. While she was in the ward the staff noted her difficulties caring for herself and taking her medication. M. told them about Miss P.'s function at home.*
>
> *At a family meeting, the medical and nursing staff told Miss P. that she should have two months in a rest home to fully convalesce. Miss P. argued but eventually agreed to one month in care.*
>
> *Once she got to the rest home, Miss P. became involved in activities and seemed to really enjoy herself. Initially she told people that she expected to go home soon, but this changed to doubt about whether she would get home at all. She never admitted that she wanted to stay at the rest home, but she made no attempt to*

> *leave. When M. visited, Miss P. would often dismiss her, saying she had other things to do, then take off down the corridor to see what was happening.*

Waiting until the person can't act on his or her desires: Sometimes people with dementia keep on saying that they want to stay in their own home, but would be unable to do anything about leaving a rest home. If taken to a rest home, they might just accept the care without being very aware of what is happening. Waiting for someone to get this disabled could put them at risk; they probably should not have been left in the community for so long. Many residential care facilities have qualms about taking in someone who is not able to agree to care, unless there is someone legally appointed to make decisions for them.

Legal Procedures (PPPR Act or MHA — see chapter 17): If someone puts themselves or others at risk because of their dementia, doctors can invoke the Mental Health Act to take that person into hospital and then, after assessment, they can be moved to a suitable rest home. The Mental Health Act is usually only used in emergency situations.

Under the Protection of Personal and Property Rights Act (PPPR Act) a judge can order someone to live at a certain place or can appoint a welfare guardian to make decisions about (among other things) where that person should live.

If a judge tells a person with dementia that they must go and live somewhere, often the person accepts this. Having the court's backing makes it legitimate for relatives to take a person to residential care, even if he or she objects. It is difficult to actually make someone go somewhere if they are refusing to move, but fortunately this doesn't seem to happen very often.

Settling in

It takes several weeks for someone with dementia to settle into a new situation. The staff of the rest home or hospital may request family not to visit for a few days while they get to know the person and the person gets familiar with the new environment. You don't have to agree to this if you believe it is better for you and your relative that you remain in close contact. If people do visit, the person with dementia may beg to be taken home, which is upsetting for everyone. If family members are agitated or upset when visiting, this communicates itself to their relative. The person's distress is not necessarily very long-lived. They may forget the visit and experienced staff can comfort and distract them.

Nevertheless, it is important to recognise their distress. Staff must pay special attention to new residents, reassuring and comforting them during the time they are adjusting to the new surroundings and routines. When they are eventually settled, it can be a great pleasure to see someone who was clearly struggling at home blossom with the good care provided in a rest home.

Life for the carer afterwards

Once their charge has gone into residential care there is an enormous void in the life of the caregiver, whether they are a spouse who has been providing 24-hour care or a daughter who visited and phoned every day. Along with the void, there may be feelings of sadness, guilt and anxiety about the sort of care being provided and the upset their relative is going through. Spoken or unspoken criticism about putting a person into a home can be hurtful and preys on the doubts and self-criticism that the carer already has. A spouse may be living alone for the first time in many decades, and the grief and loneliness can be intense. Even though their partner had severe dementia they were a physical presence, someone to hold, to talk to and share with, although there may not have been much response. Regardless of the expertise and kindness of the residential care staff, the care the person with dementia receives will initially not seem good enough, not individualised enough.

However, as the new carers get to know the person, the family will start to feel more relaxed and confident. As the person with dementia settles in, the carer's fears and doubts diminish.

It helps to have a supportive person to talk to through this period of change and doubt. As the previous caregiver takes up old hobbies and relationships, and sorts out a routine of visiting the person in care, he or she gradually comes to terms with their new lifestyle.

> *'The worst thing,' says a carer daughter, whose mother is now in a rest home, 'was the guilt. I was relieved, but I even felt guilty about feeling relieved. Every time someone asked about my mother the guilt welled up again. I am so pleased that she agreed to go into care. I would have felt terrible if I had to force her to go.'*
>
> *Asked how she got through this, she says, 'When I saw how her health improved, and when people started saying to me how well my mother looked I started to feel better. She can still make me feel guilty, but I know that she's in the best place for her right now.'*

In summary

The decision that it is time for a person with dementia to go into residential care can be a difficult and emotionally draining one. The main caregiver should get others to help choose the facility and organise the financial aspects. Although relatives sometimes feel guilty and inadequate about not managing at home, there is a limit when it is too exhausting or risky to carry on. Once the person is in residential care, the family involvement continues, as described in the next chapter.

References

[1] *Health of Older People in New Zealand: A statistical reference*, Ministry of Health, 2002.

Chapter 13

In residential care

I think of the years, all too few — gone too fast
And accept the stark fact that nothing can last
So open your eyes, nurses, open and see,
Not a crabbit old woman, look closer — see ME.

PHYLLIS MCCORMACK [1]

Many people with dementia need residential care at some stage, either in brief respite care or for a longer term. Adjusting to residential care can be difficult, but the transition can be eased if family and caregivers work together.

On admission

People being admitted to residential care are going into a strange environment and leaving familiar people and routines behind. They often feel sad, bewildered, angry, fearful or a range of other emotions. (Remember how hard it was when you first left home? And you did this voluntarily with your faculties and confidence intact.) These emotions may be expressed by changed behaviour such as increased agitation, pacing, trying to escape, aggression, withdrawal, tearfulness or clinging.

It is not always this difficult. Some people are not so aware of their environment and settle in fairly well. In other cases, the family may have been able to gradually introduce the person to the staff and the residential home, perhaps through attendance at day care or short stays in respite care. Trained caregivers know what the person is experiencing and will take the time to be reassuring and supportive. Phone calls and visits from family members sometimes help, but can also stir up feelings of loss and the desire to be home again. Familiar belongings, such as a chair, paintings or family photographs, may help the patient settle in.

No matter how good the staff, they will never be able to provide the same sort of service as a devoted family member who has given round-the-clock individual care to their relative. That is just a fact. The staff do not yet know the person with dementia, and they have others to look after as well. Relatives can get angry with residential care staff because they do not seem to be doing the very best for their family member. Some of this anger is really the relative's own grief and guilt being rechannelled at the professional caregivers. (If you are feeling guilty, you try to make it up to your family member by demanding the very best care and being angry on their behalf when care isn't perfect.) It is really important not to be too critical or suspicious of paid caregivers, but for staff and family to work together to improve the care of the person with dementia.

The family often fear that their relative will not be treated kindly. However, my overwhelming impression is that residential caregivers are kind people. They enjoy their work and get a lot of satisfaction from doing a good job. Staff are much better educated about dementia than in the past. As awareness of dementia has increased, the government has passed laws to improve the training of caregivers in dementia units and to regulate the numbers required each shift. As Tom Kitwood notes in *Dementia Revisited*, 'Most organisations involved in dementia care wish to be seen as giving excellent care; it is certainly what their "customers" desire.'[2]

Helping the staff get to know the person

Rest home or hospital staff will gather information about the new resident on admission: habits, what the person wants to be called, likes and dislikes, details of family members, friends and so on. This makes up a personal fact file. Many places make a memory book or a photo album, which tells about the important events and relationships in the new resident's past life. This means that caregivers can see the person as someone who, though now very confused, has lived a rich, full life. A memory book is also useful to provide topics of conversation. 'I see you used to ride a motor bike . . .'. It could help to decide what activities the person might enjoy, e.g., watching motorbike racing on TV (but perhaps not riding on one).

Even a small room can accommodate a few favourite pieces of furniture, a spread for the bed and pictures on the walls. A mini-CD or tape player means the resident can listen to the music they enjoy. Most people like to have their own TV. Even if the person with dementia cannot recall much, these personal touches give caregivers an indication of their tastes and history and are a starting point for getting to know them better.

Planning care

The Ministry of Health requires an initial assessment within 48 hours of admission and that a care plan be written within the first three weeks for each person being admitted. The care plan describes the help required for day-to-day functioning, medical, emotional, social and recreational needs. Usually information is gathered from the staff, the family, the new resident and any other people involved in the assessment. The written care plan is discussed with the family, who may then receive a copy. The plan states who is responsible for carrying out each part of it and when it will be reviewed. It is likely there will be many issues to deal with if the person is quite disabled. Some issues that might seem trivial, such as 'tendency to get wax in ears', might actually be very important — something like this might affect hearing and the patient would have even more trouble understanding what is said. Care plans must be reviewed six-monthly at least.

The following is a very brief care plan. In real life, there will be a lot more issues to be dealt with.

Care Plan 19 December

Mrs B. Admitted 3 December ***Diagnosis: Alzheimer's disease***

1. ***Issue*** *Occasional urinary incontinence*

Action *Remind to go to toilet before meals and at bedtime. Test for infection if urine smells or incontinence worse*

Responsible Person *Caregivers*

Review Date *3 months (18 March)*

2. Issue *Poor mobility and hip pain*

Action *Walk to meals twice daily. Physiotherapy on Mondays.* ***Observe*** *for pain and give pain relief as prescribed*

Responsible Person *Caregivers, Physiotherapist*

Review *3 months*

3. Issue *Grief over Mr B.'s death*

Action *Put photos in room. Allow Mrs B. to talk about her husband. Visit grave regularly*

Responsible Person *Daughter, Son, Caregivers*

Review *3 months*

4. Issue *Involvement with church*
Action *Take to in-house hymn singing, Thursday church services. Monthly outing to own church*
Responsible Person *Caregivers, Chaplain, Family or congregation*
Review *3 months*

There should be regular meetings with the family to review the care plan. These meetings provide an opportunity to bring up concerns about care or to give positive feedback to staff.

Over time, family members will get to know staff and start to feel confident that their relative is in good hands. There could even be times when they are a bit envious! A parent who was rude and demanding with the children may be sweet and polite with paid caregivers.

Family members, however, should not be afraid to speak up on behalf of the person with dementia if they feel that things could be done better. Hopefully communication can be calm and reasonable in both directions. Tom Kitwood expressed the responsibilities this way:

> Paid staff need to face up to the fact of being observed closely, and overcome their fear of being criticised. Family members, for their part, will need to shed their prejudices against paid staff, and appreciate how difficult their job really is; their attitude must be one of support, not disapproval. [3]

While staff provide the physical care and meet some mental health needs, the family will always be important for the person's emotional, social and spiritual needs. As the admission officer of a large care complex tells families, 'We do the caring so that you have the energy to continue the loving'. Care is not just handed over to the professionals; the family needs to remain involved.

Visiting

Visiting can be awkward if the person with dementia can't make conversation. It can be very painful for a visitor who hasn't been for a while (such as a child returning from overseas) when there has been an obvious deterioration in their relative's abilities. However, most people with dementia seem to enjoy being visited and appreciate that someone has come especially to see them.

'We keep coming and sometimes she seems to recognise us. Last week she asked me if I was the doctor,' says a devoted son-in-law who cared for his mother-in-law at home until her dementia was severe.

He keeps visiting her at the rest home because it helps reassure him to know she is well cared for. Besides, she is a delight to be with, always cheerful and laughing, even if she doesn't know who her visitor is.

Alzheimer's Australia (www.alzheimers.org.au) provided these hints for people visiting residents in care facilities:

- Ask the staff what the person's best time of day is (it's best to visit when they are not too tired) and visit then.
- Include your name in your greeting, 'Hello, it's me, Mary again' as a reminder. Don't be offended if the person doesn't recognise you. This is the result of the disease and not to be taken personally.
- Speak slowly, maintain eye contact, give the person time to respond. Talk about familiar topics so the person can contribute to the conversation.
- Bring in objects, photos or favourite flowers from the past. You can reminisce over these. Accept what may seem to be a distorted view held by the person with dementia.
- Make the person feel nurtured by helping with grooming, manicure, make-up or giving a massage.
- Read or look at newspapers, books or magazines together and discuss items of interest depending on the ability of the person with dementia.
- Play favourite card or board games if the person is still able to do so.
- Assist the person to keep in contact with friends or relatives by helping to write letters, send cards or make phone calls.
- Bring other people such as family or friends to visit. (Friends may learn from your approach and be more comfortable to come by themselves later.) Take photos while they are there so you can remind the person with dementia of the occasion.
- Encourage grandchildren and great-grandchildren to visit. Bring along something to keep the children entertained. You may have to keep visits short for young children.

- Bring in pets to visit (check first with the manager).
- Bring a special food treat, such as an ice cream (if the person has no dietary restrictions).
- Take your relative to visit another person in the facility, or go out for a walk around the grounds. Borrow a wheelchair if necessary.
- Accompany the person in any activities that are on while you're there.
- Play an instrument, sing together or by yourself; read poetry.
- Listen to music.
- Sit with your arms around the person or hold their hand.
- Keep a diary or visitor's book. This will let others know who has visited if the person forgets, and can also act as a trigger for conversation.

The end of the visit can be a difficult time, so let staff know when you are leaving so they can be available to assist.

- Let your relative know how long you can stay and what you are going to do when you leave (e.g., do the shopping, pick up children). Say when you will return. You might need to repeat this several times during the visit.
- Time your departure to coincide with an activity or meal. If there is a distraction, it makes leaving easier.
- Don't prolong the farewells, but remind the person when you will visit again.
- Remember that people with dementia have bad days, so be prepared for visits that don't go as well as you hoped. Talk to the nurse in charge if you are worried about these fluctuations.

People develop certain rituals of visiting. These are repetitive visiting patterns that include regular behaviour (such as always going for a walk) and symbolic caregiving (brushing hair, arranging flowers, etc.). Staff can accidentally discourage these rituals if they are unaware of them, but they often get to know what to expect and can prepare the person for them.

Outings

An outing could be anything from a short drive in the car to spending several days or even weeks away. When going out for a while, it is wise to check with staff first, as they may need to provide medicine, incontinence pads or a walker.

The person with dementia might enjoy going to a familiar coffee shop, for a walk in public gardens or along the beach. Some shopping malls provide wheelchairs so that frail people don't have to walk too far. Avoid going shopping during busy times when the noise and bustle will be confusing and exhausting.

Ideally a family member should take the person to outpatient clinics or doctor's appointments, as family will have the best information on the person's background. However, if that is not possible the rest home may provide transport and someone to go with the resident.

Often, the person with dementia is expected to attend important family gatherings, such as weddings, funerals, christenings and other celebrations. Most families want to include their older relatives so that they retain their place in the family. It keeps the person stimulated and aware of what is happening outside the residential care centre. However, the new environment, multiple conversations, noise, movement and greetings from people who are now unfamiliar can be very disorientating. Someone needs to keep a close eye on the person to make sure that they are neither left alone nor being overwhelmed. If possible, there should be a quiet place to withdraw to. Or the person can stay for just a short time: a brief visit and some photos with family members to remind the person later of the occasion.

Husbands and wives often like to have their spouse with dementia come home overnight on a regular basis. This gives them the opportunity for some private time together (which is difficult to achieve in the rest home). Whether this is possible depends on the carer's state of health and ability to manage and the needs of the person with dementia.

There is also no absolute restriction on taking the resident away for a holiday if the family can manage for a week or two. The residential care subsidy will continue to be paid for up to six weeks if the person is away with family. Private payers have to keep up payment for the room as long as the person still wants it, whether they are there or not.

Whenever people with dementia are away from their familiar environment they have to adjust to a new situation, both on departing and returning to care. Relatives should check whether the person was disturbed on returning to the rest home from an outing. Sometimes the distress caused by changing the person's routine outweighs the pleasure of going out, both for the person and family.

Getting other services while in residential care

People in care still need other services such as hairdressing, podiatry and dentistry. They can continue attending their usual provider in the community, though someone needs to provide transport. In most residential homes a hairdresser and podiatrist visit regularly or can be called in. Dentists and masseurs can also visit. In larger places, there will probably be regular church services. The person with dementia will need to be reminded or assisted to attend. There are usually chaplains or local religious leaders on call who can visit. There may be a small shop. There is usually transport available to take people on shopping trips if they are able to go.

Other issues

Cultural differences between residents and staff

It is often difficult for people from minority ethnic groups to fit into residential care where the staff and the other residents are mainly European New Zealanders. Language may be a real problem, as well as the strangeness of the environment. The person from the minority ethnic group may have specific religious, clothing or food requirements. They may have different ideas about care and the appropriateness of being touched by non-family members.

Although they may be angry with their family for not looking after them, it is really important that family members remain involved to communicate the needs of the person with dementia. A staff member from a similar ethnic background can help to make the resident's life happier. There are a few rest homes that cater for particular ethnic groups, and if families ask around they may find places managed or staffed by suitable people.

Many care staff (especially in Auckland) come from non-European ethnic backgrounds. There are sometimes communication difficulties, because the carer's accent is unfamiliar to the person being cared for. A person with severe dementia, who struggles to understand what is being said anyway, will find it harder if English is the caregiver's second language. It is even more difficult if the person with dementia is deaf as well!

Families should talk to the registered nurse if they feel the resident has problems with understanding a particular staff member. It may be possible to assign another caregiver or to work out other ways of communicating. A further issue is the apparent racism of some people with dementia. This can be embarrassing to the family and hurtful to staff unless they realise that the (usually) verbal abuse results from loss of inhibitions due to brain damage.

Sex and new sexual liaisons

People with dementia still have sexual needs. Husbands and wives may wish to continue their physical relationship even though one of them is living in residential care. The privacy they need is sometimes difficult to achieve within the rest home. People are always popping in to offer tea and scones. It might be necessary to explicitly ask for 'no interruptions' and to put a sign on the door to this effect. A partner (usually a wife) might not really be able to give consent to sexual activity and may not always recognise her husband. As long as she seems to be enjoying the contact, this is not a concern. However, if she seems distressed or uncomfortable after her time with her husband, the staff may need to sensitively feed this information back to him. If he persists with the physical relationship, is this considered abuse? This is a tricky issue, which can only be resolved through discussion between the staff and spouse of the person with dementia, perhaps with some input from their GP, the District Health Board staff or the Elder Abuse team.

A further, not uncommon occurrence, is that a couple in a dementia unit meet up and begin to spend time together, perhaps holding hands or getting into bed. Sometimes one or both of the couple has misidentified the other as their spouse. This can be distressing for the real spouse and some families are shocked by this out-of-character behaviour. They ask the rest home to prevent the relationship. It is hard to know whether this is the right thing to do if both people seem to like the situation.

Some families, however, accept the situation, especially when they see that it brings happiness to the person with dementia.

> *My mother was initially very restless, pacing around the rest home and always on edge. After a few months, she met a man whom she liked, and now they spend time sitting in the lounge holding hands. She seems much more settled.*
>
> *My father is happy enough too. He loves my mother, but this gives him more freedom now to continue his own life without worrying so much about her.*

The rights of the resident and family

Residential facilities should display their responsibilities and their code of patient rights. Potential residents and their families will have seen the code on admission and may wish to refer to it again. Codes will include such things as the right of the resident to:

- Have the opportunity to enhance their quality of life
- Be involved in decisions concerning them
- Make choices, unless it is clear they lack the capacity
- Have the opportunity to review their situation regularly

- Be informed of the complaints procedure (more relevant to family if dementia is advanced)
- Be assisted in retaining and exercising their citizens' rights
- Have unrestricted access to all community support services
- Have continuity in personal care and maintaining their former links
- Have private accommodation and lockable rooms
- Be shown respect for their needs and wishes, particularly with regard to religious and cultural factors
- Be treated with dignity
- Have their needs regarded as paramount by the staff
- Not be exposed to institutional practices that restrict their rights and choices
- Not have their lifestyle compromised by other activities that the home may also run (e.g., day care).

Family and friends should be able to visit the person at reasonable hours. The next of kin should be invited to care-planning meetings and to be consulted as necessary on care issues between the dates of meetings. The next of kin still has the primary responsibility for the person with dementia, even when that person is in residential care.

The Privacy Act (see chapter 17) allows the next of kin or legal guardian of a person who lacks the ability to make decisions to have access to information about that person. People with dementia who can still make some decisions should be consulted about what information the staff can give out and to whom. In practice, people with dementia are usually happy to share their details with the nearest family members. At times, though, they may refuse to allow this, especially if they are angry or paranoid. The medical staff then have to decide whether the person is competent to make a decision and how important it is to share the information. In some cases it may be necessary to go against the resident's wishes, and this is allowed for under the Privacy Act if it is necessary for the person's health.

When family or resident are not happy

The sorts of things that bother relatives range from the inconvenient to major issues of safety. Concerns should be taken to the manager or the registered nurse in charge. There is little point in complaining to primary caregivers, as they are unlikely to be in a position to change much.

People worry that if they complain, their vulnerable relative will be victimised or asked to leave. In fact, this doesn't seem to happen very often, as DHB contracts insist that residential care providers have a proper channel for complaints. Nurses and managers usually appreciate feedback, even if it is negative, as they genuinely want to provide a good service. They are used to dealing with angry or upset relatives although (as you might expect) it is better to try to approach them with an open mind and reasonable expectations.

Things getting lost or damaged

Common problems include loss of clothing or damage during washing, items going missing (such as hearing aids, glasses, dentures or jewellery), theft or loss of money or other valuables. It is better if valuables are not left with the person when they are admitted, but many people like to have a few dollars in their purse or wallet 'just in case'. They should carry only the amount they can afford to lose. If someone has precious jewellery, the family has to decide whether letting the person keep something they love is worth the risk of losing it.

Clothing should be labelled. Most facilities suggest that all clothing be machine-washable. The organisation should pay to replace damaged or lost clothing or other items if the staff have been responsible for their loss, though it is sometimes hard to tell whether the person with dementia has hidden something and forgotten where it is.

The person not being treated as an individual

To a certain extent, residents have to conform to the rules of the institution. Nursing staff also need to balance individual rights with those of other residents and the practicalities of caring for a large number of people.

Staff today are more aware of individual concerns, such as the way a person likes to have facial hair removed, the use of make-up and style of dress that are part of a person's identity. People have preferences, or religious or cultural requirements, for particular foods. There will be certain TV programmes they like to watch, bedtimes to keep to, arrangements they prefer in their rooms. If the resident is not able to complain about something, and staff don't know about or ignore their wishes, the personality of the person with dementia is further undermined, exacerbating the effects of dementia and institutional life. Families must feel free to point out what is important to the person with dementia and ask that (within reasonable limits) it is maintained. Of course, the professional caregivers might have new or better ideas, or the person with dementia may no longer desire the sort of care previously given at home. There needs to be openness and discussion around these issues.

Routines and activities

If relatives are not happy with how the person spends their day (for example, if they spend too much time just sitting around), they can discuss this with the charge nurse or manager. It may be that the person has actually been going to activities and has forgotten or is refusing to attend. The family may be able to suggest more suitable occupations or entertainment for their relative. Sometimes staff shortages or the absence of an occupational or diversional therapist is the problem. This can be taken up with management.

If the person likes to have more (or fewer) showers, more frequent hair washing or changes of clothes than they are receiving, let the staff know this and they can look at the options.

Inadequate care

If someone in care appears to have been neglected, take this up with the manager or charge nurse. Sometimes people with dementia resist caregivers who are trying to help them. This might mean a person is unshaven or not dressed when family visit and they look as if they are not being cared for properly. Often relatives can help residential care staff by explaining certain characteristics, for example, that the person is modest or embarrassed by someone of the opposite sex dealing with them. There may be a better time of the day for personal care, or a family member could come in to assist with showering and shaving their relative.

Medication and other medical issues

Many people want to be kept up to date and involved when their relative's medication is changed. If they let the registered nurse know of their interest, they can be contacted when changes are considered. When a person with dementia seems over-sedated or is suffering from other side effects, family need to bring this to the nurse's attention.

If the behaviour of the person with dementia changes, even slightly, relatives might be the first to notice and should inform staff, as the person could be in pain or have a medical problem, such as an infection. The family should ask at the next opportunity what has been done about it. Family members who are not happy with the medical management received by the resident can ask a GP or nurse to arrange for a second opinion. The cost for this will usually be the responsibility of the resident or their family.

Restraint

If a resident is restricted in some way, to stop them from doing what they want, it is known as restraint. Restraint is used to keep people with dementia safe and to prevent them hurting (usually inadvertently) others. Restraint can be environmental, that is, locked doors and fenced gardens, or physical, as in when it is made impossible for the person to move around freely, or chemical, where medication is used to sedate the person to prevent difficult behaviour.

Physical restraint includes strapping someone in a chair, placing a table in front of them to prevent them standing up, or seating them in a beanbag or armless chair that is hard to get out of. The most common form of physical restraint is 'cot sides' on the bed to prevent the person getting up at night. Studies suggest they may do more harm than good, e.g., the person gets caught between the cot side and the mattress, or falls from a greater height while climbing over them, but staff and families often feel a sense of security with them in place. It may be better for the person to have their mattress on the floor, perhaps with a pressure pad to alert staff when they get up.

There are strict guidelines regarding physical restraint and the next of kin or welfare guardian has to be consulted before it is used. This sort of restraint is difficult to use safely and is generally considered a last resort. Family can refuse to sanction the use of restraint, and accept that there is a risk to the person (usually of falls) if he or she is allowed to wander free. This should be documented in the care plan or notes. If people present a danger to others, strategies such as separating them from vulnerable residents or increasing the amount of staff observation may be a viable alternative to restraint. If there are no other feasible options, the family might want to transfer the person to another facility that manages people without using restraint.

If sedation is used as a chemical restraint and the person involved suffers ill effects, e.g., falls frequently or is overly drowsy, the family could ask the nurse whether there is another way to manage the behaviour. It may also be useful to talk to a GP about alternatives.

What if you aren't satisfied with the response to your concerns?

Take a support person: Go back and talk to the manager or registered nurse again, taking a family member or friend with you. The other person may be able to explain things in a different way, and get through where you were unable. They will help you be more assertive and can comfort you or take over if you suddenly get emotional.

Write it down: Some people find that writing a letter helps clarify their concerns. You don't necessarily have to send it. However, if words fail you in face-to face situations, writing to the management might be the best approach. Keep a copy for yourself, so you can be sure about what you said. Hopefully, at some point you will feel able to discuss the situation with the relevant person.

Involve an expert: Talk over the situation with your social worker, GP or voluntary society such as Age Concern, or your local branch of Alzheimer's

New Zealand. These people can suggest the best approach, and may talk to the rest home or hospital on your behalf. Age Concern runs the Elder Abuse Service in most areas. This may be the most relevant service to approach if you have serious concerns about what is happening.

The Health and Disability Commissioner (HDC): Rest homes and hospitals are required to display information on the HDC advocacy service so that you can contact them if necessary. An HDC advocate will help resolve the problem, or, if absolutely necessary, assist you to make a more formal complaint. The national phone line is 0800 555 050. For more information, see www.hdc.org.nz

Shifting to another place: If the worst comes to the worst, you can shift the person somewhere else. The Needs Assessment and Service Coordination (NASC) team will need to reassess the person's needs. You will have a good idea by now of their requirements and know what you are looking for. There may not be a place immediately available in your preferred rest home or hospital, in which case it will be necessary to maintain some sort of relationship with the original home while you wait. Use your family and friends to support you and to help you maintain perspective on the situation.

As the dementia progresses

People with dementia in rest homes are likely to eventually become too frail for that level of care. They will then need to be transferred to a private hospital for more intensive nursing care (after a further NASC assessment). It will be hard for both resident and family to move away from familiar faces and surroundings. Often there is a hospital on the same site as the rest home and this eases the transition a little. Usually rest homes will accommodate a person needing hospital care for a while until a bed becomes available in the preferred facility.

In summary

People with severe dementia often need residential care, but family members still have an important role to play. Professional caregivers and the family have to work together to ensure that the person in care has the best possible quality of life.

References

[1] McCormack, Phyllis: A poem found in an old lady's possesions after her death in the geriatric ward of an English hospital (www.molieb.com/crabbit.html).

[2] Kitwood, Tom, *Dementia Reconsidered: The person comes first*, Open University Press, Buckingham, 1997.

[3] Ibid.

Chapter 14
End-of-life issues

O let him pass! He hates him
That would upon the rack of this tough world
Stretch him out longer.

KING LEAR ACT V, SCENE III

Alzheimer's is a terminal disease. According to estimates from the United States, 7 per cent of all deaths result from Alzheimer's disease. This makes it the fourth leading cause of death (after heart disease, cancer and stroke).[1]

When people with advanced dementia die, it is usually from some other condition, such as pneumonia, which they develop because they are so frail. This final illness is usually reported as the main cause of death on the death certificate, but dementia may be listed as a contributing cause. Some doctors do not mention the dementia at all. This makes it difficult to work out the actual numbers of people whose death is at least partly due to dementia.

It is estimated that 32 per 100,000 people die each year as the result of dementia. In 2008 in New Zealand this equated to 1378 people.[2]

Quality of life

One man I know who was diagnosed with Alzheimer's disease said, 'When I can't read Proust any more, put me down.' I met him later, when his disease was well advanced. He was in a rest home where he sat happily in his chair with a book of Proust in front of him. He never turned the pages and sometimes the book was upside down, but he was always cheerful and the staff loved him. I knew he couldn't read anything, including Proust, but while he was still (apparently) enjoying his life so much, it seemed worth continuing on with it.

It is hard to tell in advance what we might regard as a reasonable quality of life. There are some things that we now believe are essential to our quality of life, but when we lose them later we adapt. Musicians go deaf, artists go blind, sportsmen are paralysed, professors get dementia. Generally, they adapt and carry on living fulfilling lives. Recently there have been reports of people with frontal lobe dementia developing or improving their artistic skills as they lose their speech. In an individual's overall measure of quality of life, how much does artistic ability compensate for loss of speech?

One of the difficulties about trying to give instructions on what we might want in the future is that we need to keep updating the instructions in the light of our changing circumstances. Once our ability to decide and communicate has gone, we cannot change our instructions even though they may no longer be relevant. Carers then need to decide how much notice should be taken of the previously expressed wishes of the person with dementia.

Obviously it is difficult to judge the quality of life of people who cannot tell you about it. If they appear to be able to enjoy themselves and are not too distressed, we assume that their life is satisfactory. However, once dementia is very advanced, and there is not much response to the environment or evidence of pleasure or pain, it is hard to see how prolonging life can be worthwhile.

Decisions about palliative care

The aim of palliative care is to keep patients as comfortable as possible so that they have a peaceful death, as opposed to prolonging their life through medical intervention. It is important to ensure that people who are dying can have a good relationship with their family and friends in their last days. In New Zealand, most people with dementia die at home or in residential care rather than in the public hospitals. Wherever they are, the focus should be not on extending life, but improving its quality.

Advance care planning

Early in the course of dementia, when people have the capacity to make decisions, they may make an advance care plan by writing down what sort of care they want at the end of their life. An advance care plan can either say precisely what care people want (for example, treatment for pneumonia, but not artificial feeding) or nominate a family member to make decisions for them. An advance directive is not legally binding, but the treating team should take previously stated wishes into consideration. Carrying out an advance directive may not always be possible (for example, if the person requested a lethal injection) or sensible (such as the prolongation of life by all means possible), but at least the directive gives an indication of what the person wants.

Useful information on advance care planning can be found at www.advancecareplanning.org.nz

Family decision-making

Whether the person with dementia is at home or in residential care, the family should be asked their views on treatment if it appears that their relative is close to death. The doctor should explain the options for treatment (or non-treatment) and see what the family think is appropriate and what the person with dementia might have wanted. Some families wish to have the ultimate say in what happens, but most will follow the advice of the health care team. If health professionals advise against treatment that will keep the person alive, this relieves family of any guilt they may feel about making such a momentous decision. Doctors and nurses are more used to thinking about such issues, have an understanding of the likely outcomes of treatment and are not emotionally involved, so they can gently guide the family to an acceptable solution.

At any point during the course of the illness, the family may wish to question the value of medical investigation or treatment and request that it be stopped when it seems pointless, such as treatments for high blood pressure or cholesterol that prevent heart disease in the distant future. Sometimes even quite simple treatments can be a burden to the dying person. The refusal, or stopping, of treatment is not the same as euthanasia.

Medical issues

Dehydration and poor nutrition

In the end stages of dementia, people lose the ability to swallow. This loss is part of the natural progression of the illness and will not be regained. Feeding people whose dementia has advanced to this stage is a time-consuming and difficult task. Often they choke and there is a risk they will inhale food into the lungs and develop 'aspiration' pneumonia. Carers find it very difficult when someone can neither eat nor drink, for the desire to nourish is deeply rooted in human psychology.

Sometimes doctors or families press for the administration of artificial fluids or feeding. The possibilities are:

- A nasogastric (NG) tube, down the nose through to the stomach, or
- A percutaneous endoscopic gastrostomy (PEG) tube, through the skin of the abdomen directly into the stomach.

Neither solution is perfect. Nasogastric tubes can be so uncomfortable that people struggle to pull them out and may then need physical restraint. Both PEG and nasogastric feeding still carry a risk of aspiration pneumonia because food can go back up the oesophagus from the stomach and into the lungs, especially if the person is usually lying down. These are useful procedures for people who would otherwise have a reasonable quality of life, but they are pointless if the person is already in the terminal phase of an illness. Fluids may be given by:

- An intravenous drip (fluids passed directly into the vein) or
- A subcutaneous drip (fluid is injected under the skin and is slowly absorbed into the body).

These may be used to rehydrate a patient, but they are only useful as short-term measures to allow people to make a full recovery and are not a suitable long-term answer to the problem of terminal dementia. People with dementia may accidentally or purposefully dislodge intravenous lines. Even if this doesn't happen the lines have to be replaced every few days to avoid infection, and this procedure inevitably involves some pain, or at least discomfort.

It has been suggested that dying without drinking or eating is not all that uncomfortable. The body makes its own natural opiates (pain-preventing chemicals) called endorphins that make dying relatively painless. Additional morphine can also be given to provide absolute certainty that the person is not in pain. The mouth can be kept moist with a damp swab. Death usually occurs in three to ten days if a person is not eating or drinking at all.

Pneumonia

Pneumonia is the final cause of death in many conditions. It was once known as 'the old man's friend'. Frail people lying in bed are unable to clear secretions from their chests, so fluid gathers in their lungs and becomes infected. Eventually the person cannot get enough oxygen and dies. Antibiotics can be administered to fight the infection and physiotherapy given to clear out the lungs. However, if the person's quality of life is minimal and the dementia far advanced, there is little point in vigorously working to save life. The person can be kept comfortable with morphine or a sedative if they are restless. Sometimes oxygen and suction help relieve the symptoms.

Other conditions

Pneumonia and dehydration are the usual causes of death in advanced dementia, but people with dementia can get the same fatal diseases as anyone else. For example, people with vascular dementia are prone to heart and blood vessel problems elsewhere in the body. The principles of care for these other conditions are the same: treat for comfort but avoid heroic efforts to prolong life. There is usually no need to send a person into hospital at the last moment, although sometimes admission is helpful for intensive nursing if this is not possible at home. It may be necessary to do a few blood tests or X-rays to find out how to best manage the situation, but there is no point in doing them repeatedly or investigating a potentially serious illness. Surgery is occasionally needed to control pain. When it has become difficult for the person to swallow, most of their routine medication can be stopped, leaving only that necessary for comfort. Being with someone who is dying and caring for them is more important than medical intervention.

Cardio-Pulmonary Resuscitation (CPR)

During CPR, efforts are made to restart the heart and breathing after it has stopped. This is sometimes successful in the acute situation in young people, but very rarely saves the life of someone over 70 years of age. People who do survive are often left with brain damage because the blood flow to the brain has stopped for too long. The British House of Lords, in 1994, said that CPR might be 'a traumatic and undignified interruption of the natural process of dying'. [3]

There is no place for CPR in the treatment of a person with advanced dementia.

Liverpool Care Pathway (LCP)

This system was developed to ensure the best possible end-of-life care tailored for the individual in the last few hours or days and includes social, emotional and spiritual, as well as physical, care. Many hospitals and aged residential care providers have adopted the LCP. If someone is to be placed on the LCP then the next of kin must be consulted and agreeable. More information can be found at www.lcpnz.org.nz

Euthanasia

There is a persistent interest in euthanasia in New Zealand, 'Death with Dignity' bills being introduced to Parliament every few years. The case of Rex Laws involved the 'mercy killing' of a person with Alzheimer's disease.

> *In August 2002 Rex Laws was sentenced to 18 months imprisonment for murdering his wife, who had Alzheimer's disease. He said that, 'We made a pact years ago that if any of us did get Alzheimer's, we would do each other in.' Mrs Laws had had some difficult behaviour and was not able to attend to her self-care. Mr Laws was exhausted from looking after her himself, being reluctant to accept outside help. He is described as 'a loving and devoted husband who was*

> *profoundly distressed at his wife's condition'.*
>
> *The prosecution noted that there was no evidence that Mrs Laws was suffering from physical pain, and that it was difficult to assess her quality of life. She was unable to give consent to Mr Laws' proposed course of action.*
>
> *The judge was sympathetic to Mr Laws and felt that in view of the mitigating circumstances he should impose a light sentence. He did not, however, want to send the wrong message to the community allowing 'the deliberate killing of someone suffering from such a disease or other affliction'.*

It seems difficult to tell whether or not another person's life is no longer worthwhile if that person cannot communicate. Sometimes it seems that euthanasia is advocated to reduce the suffering of family and friends, rather than that of the person with dementia. In the Netherlands, some people with dementia have undergone euthanasia, not always with an advance directive or pre-recorded request for this to occur.

People with dementia are some of the most vulnerable in our community. I believe they need protection against both 'mercy killing' and misguided attempts to prolong their lives. We need to be able to let people die naturally, but provide the best possible palliative care to support dying people and those around them.

Services available for terminal care

At home

In the final stages of a person's life, district nursing or private nursing care can be organised. Partial funding may be available to assist the family, but if 24-hour, round-the-clock care is needed, then the family will have to provide this themselves (or pay for a private nurse). There are private nursing bureaux in the larger cities, and general practitioners can help make contact, advise on what is necessary and provide medical support.

In residential care

It is more likely that people with dementia will spend their final days in a private hospital or rest home. Most hospitals are appropriately set up and have staff experienced in palliative care for older people. Often they can provide a private room if the person does not already have one. Some rest homes are reluctant to care for people who are dying, but it seems a pity at the last moment to transfer someone out of the place that has been their home. The family can discuss the possible options with the manager, perhaps offering to help or pay for additional staff themselves. If the person with dementia has had some discussion about end-of-life care or written down some of their wishes, this greatly assists in decisions about treatment. See www.advancecareplanning.org.nz

Hospices

Hospices can take people with dementia, but still tend to care for people with other diseases such as cancer or HIV/AIDs. However there is increasing interest in dementia as a terminal condition and the good palliative care of people with advanced dementia. See, for example, www.ncpc.org.uk/search/node/dementia

Spiritual and cultural needs

Hospitals and many residential homes have chaplains available to administer last rites and to support the family.

When death is pending, Maori may want to take their family member home. Whanau will wish to be present during the person's final hours and will have specific prayers and blessings to administer. After death, there are certain rituals and practices to be observed, such as the washing and dressing of the body (tupapaku), which should be respected wherever the person dies.

Bereavement

People close to the person with dementia grieve during the progression of the illness, as the loved one they knew seems to gradually fade away. Sometimes they feel that the person died a long time before their body did. This may make it easier for them to let go when, finally, the illness takes its ultimate toll. Nevertheless, most people will experience some strong emotions such as:

Numbness: feeling frozen

Denial: trouble accepting the reality of the death

Shock: even though the death has been expected

Relief and release: for the person with dementia as well as for themselves

Anger: about what has happened, both over the long term and around the death

Guilt: over any number of things, small or large

Sadness and a sense of loss

Isolation: feeling alone after the loss.

These are quite normal feelings and they generally become less intense over the next few months, though there are many conflicting feelings and marked ups and downs.

The funeral can be a time of remembering the person as he or she was.

> *I dressed him, had him in the front room. I dressed him in the last clothes he danced in. He only had a little bit of make-up on and he looked perfect. S. put photos on the wall, of his life. The kids and I spent a lot of time with him. They wrote on the lid of his coffin. I wanted him to have a can of beer in his coffin; we put a cigarette in his pocket. He had a photo of his dog and a coin in his pocket. We had him looking lovely, really.*
>
> *He was probably cursing me for making all the fuss, because he didn't like you fussing because, you know, he was a simple person.*
>
> J. SPEAKING AFTER HER HUSBAND'S DEATH

The support of friends and family is essential during this time, so you can talk through your feelings or cry and yell if need be. It is helpful to have someone around who knew the person before she or he had dementia, because they can recall the good times as well as the difficult ones.

Anniversaries, celebrations and birthdays can be sad times for a while, so make sure you plan for these. Some people like to have others around them at this time; others prefer it to be a time of solitude and reflection. It is better not to make major decisions soon after the death, as recently bereaved people may not think as clearly as usual.

It can take up to three years for the process of bereavement to run its course. Persistent, very painful feelings and difficulty coping which have not improved after two or three months may signal the development of depression. Your GP should be able to help with this. It is important for bereaved people to look after their physical as well as their mental health.

Getting on with life

There will be a huge gap in the carer's life once they have lost the person they were looking after. If the person with dementia has been cared for at home it will be hard for the caregiver to know what to do with all the time now available. No matter how disabled the person with dementia was, there was still someone there and now their absence is noticeable. Carers have often become quite isolated and may have lost contact with their friends. Perhaps they have lost confidence in social situations and now also feel they have lost their purpose in life. If the person with dementia was in residential care, the relative will have developed a pattern of visiting and have got to know the staff and other residents. This routine and social contact will now have disappeared.

Many support people, such as the hospital caregivers, doctors or Alzheimer's New Zealand, will have been involved because the bereaved person was caring for someone with dementia. Carers sometimes feel that because the person with dementia has died they can no longer 'make demands' on these support people. However, they are not expected to suddenly cut off their old contacts and make new acquaintances immediately after bereavement. In some areas, Alzheimer's New Zealand offers support groups for bereaved people, or the carer may wish to continue with the old group until they feel it is time to move on. The staff at the rest home or hospital who have got to know the family are often available for support.

Eventually, family members pick up their own lives again. They regain their confidence, the ability to make decisions and to enjoy themselves. They do not forget the last few difficult years, but those years begin to merge into a fuller picture of the person's life, with the final years only constituting a small part of that picture. One of the hard things to accept is that a person who has spent many years caring for someone with dementia may not have that time recognised by others as being useful. Another difficulty is that they may now be too old to return to the workforce.

> *Too old . . . I don't think anyone would have a 65-year-old. I'm 65 this year. Do you think you'd have me on? I'd love a job, just a couple of days a week. I don't think I could now. But probably I might end up doing something like when I was younger. I used to go and help with different organisations and things. I used to go into the crippled kids and their families in the holidays . . .*
>
> L., WHO MANAGED ROUND-THE-CLOCK CARE FOR YEARS FOR BOTH OF HER PARENTS WHO HAD DEMENTIA

Nevertheless, family caregivers are experienced, skilled and compassionate people who should be in demand for a wide range of voluntary or paid positions.

In summary

If family and health professionals communicate openly during the final phase of dementia, appropriate care can ease suffering without unnecessarily prolonging life.

It can be difficult for the bereaved caregiver to pick up and get on with life, but given time and the support of others, they can get back to living their own lives and can view the life of the person with dementia in perspective.

References

[1] Ewbank, D.C., 'Deaths attributed to Alzheimer's disease in the United States', *American Journal of Public Health*, 89: 1999, pp. 90–2.

[2] Alzheimer's NZ, Dementia Economic Report, 2008, http://tiaho.org.nz/images/uploads/docs/Economic_Impact_of_Dementia_report_2008.pdf

[3] House of Lords, BMA Guidelines on giving resuscitation to terminally ill patients — including references to BMA guide on decisions relating to Cardiopulmonary resuscitation (CPR), PQ Number 90442 Leg, 13/07/99 335c 149w.

Chapter 15

Groups with special needs

If a man does not keep pace with his companions, perhaps it is because he hears a different drummer. Let him step to the music which he hears, however measured or far away.

HENRY DAVID THOREAU

Some people with dementia do not fit into the usual patterns of illness. Services for these people may either be unavailable or unsuitable. This group includes:

- Younger people with dementia
- People with lifelong intellectual disability
- Immigrants
- People with previous serious mental illness
- Isolated individuals
- People with unusual types of dementia
- People living in rural communities.

Younger people

About 2 per cent of people with dementia are under 65 years of age. About 0.6 per cent of people aged 60–64 have dementia. Although there is a perception that there is an increased rate of young-onset dementia, this is probably due to better diagnosis and the prominence of some younger advocates. However, with the baby boomer bulge here now, we can expect an increase in the absolute numbers of 60–64 year olds with dementia.

If a younger person has dementia it is less likely to be Alzheimer's disease (34.5 per cent of younger people with dementia have Alzheimer's, compared with about 60 per cent of older people) and more likely to be due to a rare disorder (19 per cent) than in older people. The frontotemporal dementias such as Pick's or Huntington's disease are more frequent in younger people. Vascular dementia and dementia from infections or toxins (such as alcohol) may also occur in people aged less than 65.

Alzheimer's disease that develops early in life sometimes runs in families.

For people developing dementia at a younger age, there may be an advantage in seeking genetic counselling to see if there are hereditability issues. If there is a genetic link, other family members can be alerted in case they want to be tested too. Some people in this situation will want to find out if they have an increased risk of Alzheimer's disease; others would prefer not to know. (See chapter 2 for more on the genetics of Alzheimer's.)

Assessment

Because many doctors don't expect a younger person to have dementia, and also because they may present with an unusual form of dementia, it is more difficult to diagnose. Younger people may have to see several doctors and try various forms of treatment before the correct diagnosis is made. This is unfortunate, as dementia tends to progress faster in younger people.

In New Zealand, younger people with memory problems are likely to be referred to a neurologist for investigation. There can be a long wait for a hospital outpatient appointment if the person cannot afford to attend a specialist in private. Getting tests done, especially brain scans, can mean a further delay. All this can be immensely frustrating and worrying. Private health insurance often covers both specialist assessment and scans, so it is worth enquiring about going privately if the person suspected of having dementia has a health insurance policy.

Work

Most younger people with dementia are still in employment when the diagnosis is made. As well as the obvious need to earn a living for themselves and their families, work is a source of satisfaction and self-esteem. It is hard for people with dementia to give up working. However, it is essential that they do not endanger themselves or others because of the illness. They may need to move to a more suitable job or adapt the current one to their changed circumstances. At some point, they will have to inform their employer of the diagnosis and perhaps their co-workers too, so they can make any necessary job changes and hopefully receive their support.

The story below demonstrates the difficulties of being diagnosed with dementia and continuing work.

> *In her 50s, Mrs E. was working in a responsible position registering and inspecting childcare providers and playgroups. She was a very active and creative person who enjoyed travelling with her husband.*
>
> *When major changes were introduced to her job she found it difficult to cope, but put this down to her older age. Mr E. became*

aware that she had memory problems when she forgot to peel the potatoes one night for dinner.

They went to the doctor who told them that her symptoms were due to 'pressure of work', so she decided to go part time. However, when she got lost driving, it was clear then that she could not manage her job, which required her to visit the various childcare centres. She retired early.

Mr E. took voluntary retirement himself. He wanted to spend as much quality time with his wife as possible. They managed to go on a couple of overseas trips, which they both enjoyed.

The diagnosis is important if someone with dementia needs to retire early. They may be able to receive their pension (although sometimes at a reduced rate) or be eligible for disability insurance payments through the organisation for which they work. Self-employed people often have private disability insurance that may be paid once the diagnosis is made. Sometimes employers or insurance companies do not believe that a younger person could have dementia. In this case it would be necessary to get a letter from the diagnosing GP and specialist doctor and perhaps be seen by a doctor employed by the insurance company. This could take a long time and is likely to be distressing for the person with dementia and their family, who will already be distraught about the diagnosis. The Human Rights Commission may be able to help people who suspect they are being discriminated against because of disability, i.e. dementia (or because of their age). Phone: 0800 496 877, www.hrc.co.nz

Family

Younger people with dementia may have children living at home. They will probably be teenagers, though they could still be quite young. (The following applies to grandchildren as well.) Children of any age need to understand what is happening. They need to know that their relative's change in behaviour and personality is caused by an illness and not directed at them. They need to know it is not their fault. Explanations about the illness may have to be repeated on several occasions and in different ways. If children are still at school, it is a good idea to inform the head teacher of what is happening.

Children react in a variety of ways. Older children may feel that they have to take over and do the things that the parent with dementia can no longer do. They might be angry, because this added responsibility eats into their own time, or anxious because they don't feel able to take over the parent's role properly. They are often embarrassed by an ill parent and are almost always sad. Teenagers sometimes 'act out' by taking risks or retreat to their bedrooms and avoid social contact. They also have to deal with the grief of losing the attention and involvement of a parent, who while physically present may not always be fully aware of important events in the child's life, such as graduation or getting their first job. Teenagers may also be concerned about the risk of inheriting dementia.

The situation can be very difficult for spouses, who have to cope with their own feelings about what is happening and take on tasks that the partner can no longer perform, as well as being physically and emotionally available to the younger members of the family.

Some suggestions for dealing with younger people:

- Listen to what children have to say and encourage them to ask questions so you can find out what is worrying them.
- Use examples of things that have happened (e.g., forgetting things or getting lost) to help the young person get a clearer idea of how the illness affects their parent.
- Use humour when possible.
- Try to make sure that time spent with the person with dementia is pleasurable. You may be able to think of shared activities both can enjoy.
- Emphasise that just being with the person and showing love is the most important thing they can do.
- Don't leave children alone with the person with dementia unless you are certain that they are happy with this and are able to cope with any situation that might arise.
- Don't overburden children or expect them to take on roles that they are not mature enough for.
- Give reassurance and cuddles and try to be available or have another family member who can support the child.
- Let children know how much you appreciate their help and love them.

Websites with resources for children are listed at the back of the book.

Services

Younger people with dementia fall between different services; they are not old enough for the over-65 services but don't necessarily fit in with disabled younger people, such as those with brain damage or psychiatric illness. This means that it might be hard to find suitable help for them. Needs assessment services for people under 65 (which are different from the NASC service for people over 65) should be able to arrange ongoing support, though this is usually the same as that provided for people over 65. Some geriatricians or old-age psychiatry teams treat younger people with dementia. The day care and respite services available for younger people are the same as those used by older people.

Many younger people are not happy being put with elderly folk and prefer to be with their own age group.

> *He picked up that there were a lot of old people around him and I find that hard, because there is nowhere they have a place for young Alzheimer's sufferers. When you think about it, the music they play in the old people's home is not from his era. J.'s era should be 60s and 70s music.*
>
> WIFE TALKING ABOUT CARE FOR HER 60-YEAR-OLD HUSBAND AT DAY CARE

In some countries, services specifically for younger people with dementia are being developed. Workers in these services become expert at managing the particular issues that concern this age group (like dealing with work and children) and also at getting suitable support for their patients. In this country, Alzheimer's New Zealand is advocating for a better deal for younger people with dementia and ideally with specialist services just for them, but even in the larger cities the number of people or the distances between them make this difficult.

Finances and benefits

People in their forties or fifties are likely to still be funding their children's education or paying off a mortgage. Developing dementia when they are about to begin saving for retirement can be very difficult. Partners may continue to work, but eventually may have to stop to become a caregiver. This can be a hard decision, especially if they had good chances of promotion and increased pay, or even if they just liked their work.

People with dementia are entitled to an Invalid's Benefit. The amount varies according to the number of dependents, and there are additional payments for other services such as doctor's visits, drugs, day care, etc., but it can still be hard to make ends meet. The Invalid's Benefit is means-tested, taking into account income but not assets. If the spouse or partner is still working, this reduces the amount paid in the benefit.

> *He got no money off the government, it makes you laugh, it makes you angry too. You work all your life and don't get a penny off the government.*
>
> *Because I was earning they wouldn't give him anything, but I can tell you now, they paid for care . . . we didn't have to pay for that, have to be grateful for that . . . the respite, they paid for that and towards the end I could get as much as I wanted.*
>
> J., WHO CONTINUED WORKING AFTER HER HUSBAND DEVELOPED ALZHEIMER'S DISEASE AT 55

The partner who stays home to care for someone with dementia may be eligible for the Domestic Purposes Benefit. Both partners qualify for the government pension, the guaranteed retirement income (GRI), once they turn 65. Residential care is not asset-tested for people under 65. Check what you are entitled to with your local WINZ office.

Behavioural and emotional problems

Younger people are stronger and healthier physically than older people with dementia. This means that they may continue to enjoy physical activities once intellectual ones become too challenging. However, if there are behavioural difficulties, it is harder for others to control the person and they can do more damage. If the person is in residential care with frail older people they may be a danger to them.

Younger people have not had to accept the inevitable slowing down that occurs with greater age. They still expect to be able to do what they want and will become frustrated when they can't. This frustration can show up in difficult behaviour.

> *It has been difficult for Mr E. to find suitable day care for his wife, in her early 60s, who has become very restless, often agitated or pacing. She is still physically strong and it is hard to get her to do what you want. If she wants to lie down on the floor, she does. When trying to sit down, she often misses the seat and won't let people redirect her.*

She is now receiving day care with older people, but as Mr E. says, 'She doesn't fit into a pigeon hole . . . a category.'

She will soon need 24-hour nursing care. Mr E. has found a place that seems suitable, though he will have to wait for a vacancy. He thinks that she is probably not very aware of her surroundings any more and it won't matter too much at this stage if she is with older people.

Younger people may still be sexually active, which might be difficult for a partner who no longer feels able to communicate on an intimate level. Or the person with dementia may lose interest in sex altogether and their spouse will have to cope with this.

Driving

Driving is an important symbol of independence and it may be very difficult for younger people to give up this activity (see chapter 17). It can also put a major burden on the family if the person with dementia is unable to do their usual chores because they can no longer drive safely.

People with intellectual disability

The commonest cause of lifelong intellectual disability (ID) is Down's syndrome. This is usually (though not always) caused by problems with chromosome 21, one of the chromosomes thought also to be involved in Alzheimer's disease. A large proportion of people with Down's syndrome develop an Alzheimer-like dementia by middle age or earlier: about 55 per cent are afflicted by the time they reach 60–69 years of age.

It is not yet entirely clear whether people with other sorts of intellectual disability are more prone to developing dementia. (Some research suggests they are about four times more likely to get dementia than the general population.) However, what is known is that as more and more people with ID are living to old age, we can expect more of them to develop dementia.

Diagnosis

It can be difficult for someone who does not know the person with ID to make a diagnosis of dementia. A doctor making a one-off assessment may be confused because the person with ID already has a range of memory, thinking and judgement problems and it will be hard to tell which of these have always been there. People with ID may have difficulty explaining their symptoms. The usual tests, such as the MMSE or MOCA (see chapter 3), will not be helpful unless they have been taken earlier and repeat testing yields a lower score. There are now diagnostic tests specifically for people with intellectual disability, e.g., the Dementia Screening Questionnaire for Individuals with Intellectual Disability (DSQIID). For these tests the carer is asked questions about the person with intellectual disability. This caregiver or family member will be able to describe what the person with ID was previously like and what they could normally do. They will be able to say whether there have been changes in behaviour and if skills have been lost. Often they describe situations where the person's memory is not what it used to be, for example, forgetting the names of people who are familiar. Nevertheless, it is still sometimes difficult to tell what is going on.

Miss A., a lady with Down's syndrome, became frightened of going into small places, such as the toilet or shower.

A psychological programme and medication to reduce her anxiety helped a little, but eventually she stopped being able to cope in other situations as well.

Along with various other tests, a CT scan was performed. This showed severe brain shrinkage.

Belatedly, we realised that her fear of small spaces was because she had difficulty in judging distance and depth, which can occur early in Alzheimer's disease. She was frightened of going into places that must have seemed too small or as if they were crowding in on her.

It is important that the person is fully investigated, in case there are medical problems that can be remedied. For example, reduced thyroid function (hypothyroidism) is common in people with Down's syndrome, and once treated their cognitive abilities may improve. People with ID can also develop mental illness, such as depression, which interferes with their usual lives and activities. Once treated, they may return to normal.

Services

It is sometimes hard to find the right health service to assess and treat people with intellectual disability and dementia, especially if they are aged less than 65 years. Mental health teams for adults are not experts in intellectual disability and old-age teams might not want to take on younger people. The need for dementia services in the intellectual disability field is now being recognised. In many areas there are specialist teams that treat people who have both intellectual disability and mental illness, including dementia. Otherwise, an older people's service may see such patients, even if they are less than 65 years of age.

People with ID may be living at home with their family, in supported housing provided by a non-governmental organisation or, sometimes, in a rest home. Some live in 'sheltered villages', where several houses are grouped together and there are day programmes, workshops and recreational facilities for the residents. If an organisation manages several houses or a village, people with dementia can live together in a house with specially trained staff. However, people with ID who develop dementia will still need to be transferred to mainstream rest homes or private hospitals when they need more intensive care than their own home can supply.

Treatment

The principles of treatment are just the same as for other people with dementia. People with intellectual disability and dementia need help to maintain their skills and self-esteem, without being pushed so hard that they become anxious or frustrated — it's a delicate balance. If someone always had limited means of communication or expressed themselves through their behavioural patterns, then this will continue once dementia develops. If their behaviour changes abruptly, then the carer needs to look for the cause, which may lie in the living situation (including changes in relationships with others), or physical or mental illness. Family and care staff are often already experts at doing this. If there are behaviour problems that can't be managed in any other way, then the medications listed in chapter 9 can be used — with caution. A very useful programme is 'Supporting Derek', available for a small amount at www.jrf.org.uk/publications/supporting-derek

ACEIs (the anti-dementia drugs) may help people with the dementia associated with Down's syndrome. There is no reason not to try this medication especially now that donepezil is funded.

People with long-standing mental illness

Schizophrenia

People with long-standing mental illness are not more likely than anyone else to get dementia, but people with chronic schizophrenia can develop frontal lobe problems that result in poor motivation, odd behaviours and lack of social awareness. Emil Kraeplin, the psychologist who first described schizophrenia, recognised this when he named the disease 'dementia praecox' (praecox means 'early onset'). The behavioural pattern seems to be the combined result of having a serious brain disease, spending long periods in the restrictive environments of a mental hospital and the side effects of the drugs used to treat schizophrenia. Now that people with schizophrenia can get modern treatment and are not placed in mental hospitals long term, cognitive deterioration may be less of a problem.

Other mental illnesses

There is a suspicion that people with recurrent episodes of depression or those developing depression late in life may have a higher rate of dementia. Alcohol and drug abuse cause brain damage. The damage may reverse to some extent if the person stops using alcohol or drugs, but stopping is the hard part. People with lifelong anxiety will find their symptoms worsen as cognition deteriorates.

Diagnosis

People with chronic mental illness, especially in the older age group, are sometimes isolated from family and society. They may develop memory problems without anyone noticing or have unusual behaviour ascribed to mental illness. They are thus less likely to be seen early in the course of dementia. Often they are suspicious of doctors (perhaps having had a difficult relationship with them earlier in life) or may not wish to use their limited funds to pay for a consultation. If a general practitioner or specialist team can visit the person at home, this overcomes the practical problem of getting the patient to a doctor. The clinical team often needs to work hard to develop a positive relationship with the person.

It can be hard to tell whether odd speech and poor self-care relate to the long-term illness or a developing dementia. Making the diagnosis can be difficult because of the cognitive changes associated with schizophrenia (one study found that about 60 per cent of people with chronic schizophrenia had an MMSE of less than 24). Often there is no one who has known the person long enough to give a good account of recent changes. Sometimes the psychiatric team has to treat the mental illness and then wait and watch to see if the patient's memory declines over time, in order to confirm a diagnosis of dementia.

Treatment

Untreated mental illness of any type (schizophrenia, depression, alcohol dependence) will interfere with a person's ability to think and will make the effects of dementia worse. The mental illness needs to be managed as well as possible and attention should also be paid to the patient's physical health. People may need careful supervision to make sure they take their medicine as directed and that they care for themselves adequately. Very intensive care is usually beyond the scope of a GP and requires the input of the community mental health team and other support services.

As the dementia progresses, or if it is impossible to care for them in the community, these patients may need to go into residential care. People with long-term mental illness sometimes seem eccentric and tend not to fit easily into the average rest home. It is sometimes hard to find the right place.

Immigrants

Each group of immigrants comprises different regional groups, arriving at different times, for different reasons, at different ages, with different levels of education, English language and 'Westernisation'. Sometimes they have fled from frightening circumstances. Others have been able to make a more considered decision to allow their move. Moving to a new country when you are older is difficult. The person has to adjust to a new climate and culture, another language and a different role. Sometimes the older person is brought over to care for grandchildren while the parents work to get established in their new country. Older people can be isolated if they do not speak English and do not have contact with others from their own country. Their children may have adopted New Zealand customs and be less interested in remembering the country they left behind.

As dementia progresses, people tend to lose their second language first (in this case English) and revert to their native tongue, which makes communication (and diagnosis) even more difficult. People with dementia will feel increasingly alienated as they lose their English and will remember less and less about their current home and begin to live more in the past. Refugees may relive desperate times from earlier in their lives, as their memory for the present diminishes. They will often feel very alone and frightened and will need reassurance from someone who knows their background and can speak their language.

Many immigrant groups have social clubs, but people with dementia will not necessarily be able to cope with these. There are interpreting services available in the public health system and there are also home help and residential services for older people of specific ethnic groups. For example, there is a Dutch residential village in West Auckland. (There is more about different cultural groups in chapter 16.)

People who are isolated

There are people in our neighbourhoods who appear to have no family or anyone who takes an interest in them. They may have neighbours, acquaintances at church or in the shops, but no obvious close friends or relatives. They might have a GP, but neighbours probably wouldn't know who that was. It is really difficult to decide who should take action if something seems to be wrong, and also difficult to know when and how to approach the person.

People are usually isolated for a reason. Perhaps all their close relatives have died or moved away. Perhaps they somehow alienated people who were once close. Neighbours who try to get involved might be told sharply to 'mind your own business'. Yet those neighbours would probably feel terrible if the person burned the house down or spent nights on the floor after falling. They might also become concerned if they noticed the person behaving oddly or neglecting him- or herself.

A possible course of action might be to:

- Approach the person and offer help, perhaps taking a friend or neighbour with you. If you are rebuffed at first, but have the time and persistence, try again, perhaps at different times of the day.
- Try to discover the name of the person's GP (or one of their relatives), and ask if you can phone them. Even if permission is not granted, if you are really concerned, you should go over the person's head and do it anyway.
- If you can't get any information and are still concerned, contact any local GP, the police (especially if the person is at risk), Alzheimer's New Zealand, a social worker from the local hospital's older people's service, or the mental health team.

Neighbours in a block of flats notified the Old Age Service when Ms V. was seen on several occasions in her dressing gown waiting at her letterbox or walking down the street. They were concerned that she would get cold or be harmed.

The geriatrician visited and persuaded Ms V. to let him in. He found the house cluttered with multiple purchases, including unpacked bags of old groceries. She had been paying a taxi driver to get her shopping, but had no idea what things cost or what to do with them.

Among the clutter, the geriatrician found the name of one of Ms V.'s friends. Later, a social worker tracked the friend down. The friend had, in fact, been keeping an eye on Ms V., but had never been able to persuade her to accept other help. She still couldn't, but the friend met the neighbours so they knew whom to contact if they were concerned. She made arrangements to pay the taxi driver a reasonable amount to get suitable shopping and put it away. The geriatrician was able to confirm that Ms V. was suffering from dementia and checked her physical health.

With these arrangements in place, Ms V. managed to stay another year in her flat.

Unusual types of dementia

There are over seventy different types of dementia. I have focused only on the common ones in this book. Most doctors know about Alzheimer's disease or vascular dementia, but the others may be a bit of a mystery to them.

Diagnosis

The unusual types of dementia are more difficult to recognise because most doctors will not have had experience with them. They may not start with memory loss. They are often misdiagnosed and treated as something else, or the person may be dismissed as being a hypochondriac. People who are concerned that their own or their relative's illness has not been properly diagnosed or treated should ask their doctor to arrange for another opinion. Usually people who have these unusual disorders have to be referred to specialist services such as a neurologist or a memory clinic for diagnosis and treatment.

In some diseases, such as Huntington's disease, Parkinson's disease or HIV/AIDS, dementia is a known problem and doctors and relatives will be on the lookout for symptoms suggesting dementia. Rather than being missed, the dementia may be anticipated.

Services

People with the rarer forms of dementia may feel even more isolated than others with dementia. Nevertheless, they can still gain support from their local Alzheimer's group. They may also find the Internet useful for getting more information about their particular form of illness and linking into support networks in New Zealand and overseas. In most areas, there may be additional support from other agencies such as the Huntington's Disease Society. Many people will already be involved with such groups before the dementia becomes evident.

The standard services are available, though they are not always entirely suitable if the person with dementia is younger or shows unusual behaviour. If the person needs to go into care it is very helpful for the staff to have some information about the illness. If the family can provide written material, perhaps provided by a medical specialist or a reputable Internet source, the staff are likely to be both interested and grateful.

People living in rural communities

People living in the country may have difficulty accessing services, both for diagnosis and ongoing care. They may be worried about managing the farm. A family farm, intended for the next generation, may be lost if the person is asset-tested as part of the move into residential care.

Diagnosis

In areas not too distant from old-age medical and psychiatric services, a nurse or doctor can make a home visit for the first assessment. However, often the person with dementia and the family need to make several long trips to a city hospital to confirm the diagnosis. There are still some areas of New Zealand that lack a regional geriatric or psychogeriatric service, and neurologists are rarely found outside the main centres, though they sometimes visit smaller hospitals.

Services

It may be difficult for rural patients to get ongoing in-home care and be too far for them to travel to support groups. The person with dementia and the caregiver could end up isolated, unable to make contact with neighbours and having only erratic input from support services. This is compounded if the partner of a person with dementia does not drive. The local district nurse or GP, neither of whom will necessarily have specialised knowledge about dementia, may be the main professional support in this case.

It can be difficult to get help in the home. Needs Assessment and Service Coordination (NASC, see chapter 11) will approve funding for help to be given by relatives or local people who are available, even if they are not part of an organisation or bureau contracted to provide care. It may still be difficult to find a suitable person in a sparsely populated region, but it would be worth contacting the Country Women's Institute, as they can sometimes help out.

If the person with dementia needs residential care, it is likely to be a long way from home. This is particularly so if the person needs specialist dementia care, as such rest homes and hospitals are few and far between. The family will have to make the difficult choice between visiting their relative less often or moving into town to be close to them.

In summary

Younger people who develop dementia do not always fit in well with older people who have dementia. They often have the more unusual forms of dementia, which are difficult to diagnose. People with intellectual disability also pose diagnostic dilemmas. ID service providers know their population is ageing and are beginning to plan accordingly. People with long-standing mental illness and dementia present challenges in diagnosis and care. As people of different ethnic backgrounds immigrate and age we are becoming more aware of their needs, though we are a long way off providing ideal care. People isolated by habit or geography may be difficult to assist.

Chapter 16

Spiritual and cultural issues

Human life under any circumstances never ceases to have a meaning, and this infinite meaning of life includes suffering and dying, privation and death.

VICTOR FRANKL [1]

In Western society, two really important values are autonomy — the ability and freedom to make our own decisions — and self-reliance or independence — not having to rely on others, not being a burden. Associated with autonomy and independence is the concept of identity — deciding and acting for oneself gives the individual a unique identity. Decision-making and independent action require a well-functioning brain. Losing these abilities, and hence one's identity, makes dementia a much-feared condition.

However, even when well, none of us are entirely autonomous. Unless we are hermits, we are bound to take account of other people's needs and feelings. We don't really value people who ruthlessly assert themselves regardless of others. The women of the current older generation often did not have much autonomy. They sometimes had very little say in important aspects of their lives and only managed to get their way by subtle manipulation of their menfolk, rather than the direct expression of their wishes.

It is also impossible to live in society without being reliant on others, in some way or other. We depend on the government for roads, our lawyers for advice, our families for emotional support, our friends for companionship, our lovers for sexual satisfaction and so on.

> Absolute independence is a false idea. It delivers not the autonomy it promises, but loneliness and vulnerability instead.
>
> ROBERT BELLAH [2]

Our fears of being dependent on others reflect our lack of trust. We find it hard to believe that people will treat us kindly if we have to rely on them. We fear being hurt, neglected, exploited, demeaned and abused. We think we will lose our dignity. We are afraid we will just be treated as one of a number and our uniqueness as individuals will not be recognised. These fears are based on history. It is not long since Victorian times when older people who were unable to look after themselves lived in the workhouse, where they survived, but in humiliating circumstances. Until recently, in New Zealand, people with dementia often spent their last days in big mental hospitals where they were fed and clothed, but where their individual needs could not be met. These institutions have only just closed down. How can we be sure that things have changed?

Are people with severe dementia still people?

Many people consider dementia such a devastating disorder because they believe someone with Alzheimer's disease loses their identity and becomes a 'non-person' or 'disappears'. Many carers describe their family member as having 'gone'. They say such things as 'This is not the woman I married . . .' or 'He's just a shell . . .' .

> *At his father's trial, Rex Laws' son said, 'I never had a mother for the last few years . . . She didn't recognise any of us . . .'*
>
> REX LAWS KILLED HIS WIFE WHO HAD ADVANCED DEMENTIA

It feels as if, though the person with dementia is still physically present, their mind has died and the spirit has gone away. This is a terribly painful situation for a family member who has lived with, loved and cared for someone for years.

On the other hand, sometimes people catch a brief glimpse of the person they once knew. The face of the person with dementia suddenly lights up listening to an old tune, or the person tenderly strokes the head of a child they no longer recognise as a granddaughter. These glimpses can be even more heartbreaking; they are sudden reminders of what is lost.

> *He had this wonderful sense of humour and would get this twinkle in his eye. You would see he would just focus on her and then all of a sudden his eyes were really alive.*
>
> L., TALKING ABOUT HER FATHER WITH ADVANCED ALZHEIMER'S DISEASE

When we think a person with dementia has ceased to be a person, this is often because we focus on those attributes they have lost: autonomy, independence (and economic productivity and intellectual ability). We are not acknowledging what the person might have contributed in the past, their importance as members of a family or whanau, their ability to love and be loved and, in their own way, to teach us. If we deny these aspects and judge people with dementia only on their ability to be independent, thinking beings, then we will begin to think of them as non-people.

Maori have a more holistic view of health, acknowledging physical, spiritual, family and mental wellbeing as essential ingredients. They do not value intellectual abilities above all others and do not regard autonomy and self-reliance as necessarily healthy. In Maoridom, even if people develop dementia, they are still important because of their place in the community, in the past and future as well as the present.

Tom Kitwood writes:

> Above all else, the reconsideration of dementia invites us to a fresh understanding of what it is to be a person. The prevailing emphasis on individuality and autonomy is called into question, and our true interdependence comes to light. Frailty, finitude, dying and death are rendered more acceptable; grandiose hopes for technical Utopias are cut to the ground. Reason is taken off the pedestal that it has occupied so unjustifiably, and for so long; we reclaim our nature as sentient and social human beings. Thus from what might have seemed the most unlikely quarter, there may yet emerge a well-spring of energy and compassion. [3]

Why does it matter whether people with dementia are still people?

It matters that people with dementia are still people (and not 'shells' or 'empty bodies') on a number of fronts.

- It seems vital to do all that we can to help retain a person's individuality, to help them be themselves for as long as possible. We hate the thought of our own personal extinction at death. What must it be like to feel yourself slipping away while you're still alive? Anticipating these changes in herself, Christine Boden, who had dementia, called her book *Who will I be when I die?* Maintaining someone with dementia's 'personhood' is not only a compassionate thing to do, but also perhaps the main goal of care.
- If people, even in the late stages of dementia, are seen as people then we are obliged to care for them in the best manner possible. We should make treatment available to improve their quality of life. Their caregivers should be well supported, trained and paid adequately.
- We have to take account of their wishes, previously and currently

expressed. They deserve to have adequate services to allow them to stay at home if that is what they want. We might develop alternative forms of residential care. We could let people with dementia sleep all day and walk all night if they felt like it. We would tolerate a dirty house and let the cleaner spend her time chatting and looking at old photos. We would keep them comfortable, but not force treatment on them to keep them alive.

- If people with dementia are seen as people we cannot do to them things that we would not do to other members of the public. We cannot lock them up without consent, unless a Court of Law allowed this. We cannot tie them to chairs or give them drugs to limit their freedom of movement or expression without legal backing. We cannot euthanase them. We have to acknowledge their human rights. To not do so leaves very vulnerable people open to abuse.

Spirituality

In this book, spirituality is defined as whatever gives meaning to people's lives. It is whatever makes someone truly human and it recognises the difference between individuals. Spirituality may be expressed via a religion, but could involve other concepts such as beauty, love of friends or family, or a broad notion of God that is not attached to any particular system of belief. Throughout life, people imbue events with their own meaning and develop their own spirituality. Different cultures have different ideas of what is ultimately important. Frail elderly people have to cope with a sense of hopelessness and uselessness, loss of identity, the fear of dying and being alone when dying, and dependence on others for very intimate care. Spirituality brings hope and comfort even in these most difficult of times.

How do people with dementia manage to retain their spiritual integrity so that they can still have hope and find meaning in life? Early in the course of her illness Christine Boden wrote: 'I shared with her one of my main worries . . . that I would lose my awareness of God before I die.'[4]

As the capacity to make and act on their own wishes fades, it can be very difficult for people to hold on to concepts that give their life meaning. This is especially true if people are in a situation where little regard is paid to their individual needs.

The following factors contribute to an inability to retain the spiritual aspect of life:

- Difficulty with memory and thinking, loss of initiative

- Psychological problems such as depression or delusions (false beliefs) which affect hope and understanding of one's situation
- Trouble coping with social demands, such as going to a church service
- Loss of awareness of God, feeling purposeless and valueless
- Other physical disabilities such as deafness, difficulty understanding words, transport problems, poor energy.

It is no surprise that people can come to feel lost and disconnected from everything that matters to them. When they can no longer do what is necessary to keep their spirituality alive, others need to assist, just as much as they help with practical things such as dressing and showering.

Reconnecting to spiritual life

Religion and culture

The use of ritual: Many symbols and rituals give meaning to life: familiar patterns of worship, the traditions of the marae, prayer beads, readings from the Bible, the Koran or other books of worship. When words are lost, significant objects or actions help people connect to something beyond themselves.

Sharing with others involved in the same rituals or festivals: Attending services with others generates a sense of belonging. If people cannot get to church in the flesh, they can watch a TV programme such as *Praise Be* or listen to radio broadcasts of religious services. Some innovative churches provide a DVD or audio tape of Sunday services.

Prayer: Often people with dementia can remember the words of set prayers, or can say them along with someone else. 'In prayer I get muddled or vague, wandering off . . . So I find using the Prayer Book daily services is one way of really helping me focus my time with God.'[5] Even when people with dementia cannot say the words, listening to someone else saying them can be comforting.

Readings: Reading religious writings, meaningful poetry or meditations (or having them read) will help people stay in contact with their spirituality. It is important that the language is right for older people. Readings from the Good News Bible will be unfamiliar to someone who only remembers the King James Version from their childhood.

Maintaining cultural links: Recognising a person's culture helps reinforce that they are part of a society that gives place and meaning to their lives. As dementia progresses they may only remember the traditional patterns of life in their youth. To maintain cultural links people have specific language, dress, food and religious requirements. They need ongoing involvement with people from their own culture, especially those who can speak in their native tongue as they lose their mastery of English. This can be difficult if the younger generation has adopted the culture of their new home.

Sharing with others

Reminiscence: Life review is something that older people do whether they have dementia or not. Having people with dementia tell their story helps make meaning of their lives. A sympathetic listener can share the celebration of great events and help people forgive themselves if they feel guilty. The listener could be a family member, a nurse or counsellor, a kaumatua or minister. The listener benefits as well, receiving the wisdom of older people. A useful book, *Facilitating spiritual reminiscence for older people with dementia — a learning package*, by Elizabeth MacKinlay and Corinne Trevitt (2006) is available via http://www.centreforageing.org.au/html/publications.htm

Talking about death: Older people need to come to terms with death and might want to talk about dying. Family and other carers sometimes want to avoid the topic, as they are uncomfortable with it. It may be difficult for people with dementia to fully express their feelings in words, but perhaps it is only necessary that someone sits with them and tries to understand. If this is too hard, a kaumatua, religious leader or counsellor will be able to fill this role.

Expressions of love: It is sometimes hard to hug someone who doesn't recognise you or has food on their clothing. Yet people with dementia have the same need as everyone else for physical affection, perhaps more so if other means of giving and receiving love have gone.

> *He could never put his arms around you, so you had to give him a cuddle and then it would click, and he would give you a cuddle, but he didn't know how to do it because of the illness.*

Contact with family and friends: Remaining in contact with old friends and colleagues reassures people with dementia of their place in society and reminds them what they have given to society. Seeing grandchildren, former students, old friends or caregivers reassures them that they have been and still are important to many people.

Keeping people involved in what matters to them

Music: Music speaks directly to the emotions and the soul. It can be comforting or exhilarating. Music lovers will have their own favourites; some find depth in the words of old hymns. Astonishingly, people who haven't spoken a word for months can join in a sing-along with familiar songs. Dancing is another age-old way of expressing emotion and meaning.

> *I used to play all kinds of music, but usually classical music. I bought a player for the bedroom and put on the music and Dad loved the music, just loved it . . .*

Keeping in touch with nature: Taking people out to enjoy the garden or look at the sunset will help maintain a sense of peace, awe or oneness with the world, even if they have no words to describe it. (People without dementia don't either.)

Art, architecture: People may still love looking at beautiful pictures or being in places with inspiring architecture. They often still enjoy painting late in the course of their illness. They may feel freer to express themselves creatively as the dementia makes them less inhibited.

Sport: If sport is a lifelong interest then backing a team and being caught up in the enthusiasm around special events can give someone a sense of meaning and belonging.

The spiritual, emotional, social and physical wellbeing of people with dementia can be seen when they are able to assert their will, express emotion, make social contact, be affectionate, accept other people with dementia, be socially sensitive, show self-respect, have a sense of humour, show pleasure, be creative, helpful and be able to relax.[6]

Cultural issues

Acknowledgement of cultural differences is important if people are to retain their identity. Healthcare workers are much more aware of these differences than they used to be, but there is still a long way to go to meet various cultural needs in dementia care. In any group, regardless of the overall culture, there will be an enormous range of attitudes, education and incorporation of New Zealand Pakeha values. Any comments about a particular culture have to be very general and I have mainly focused on differences from mainstream ideas.

Maori

Life expectancy in Maori is significantly lower than for European New Zealanders. On average, Maori men can expect to live to 70.4 years of age (compared to 79 years for their European counterparts), Maori women to 75.1 years (83 years for European New Zealand women). At present only 4 per cent of Maori are over 65 years old.[7] Because fewer Maori live to old age there is less chance of them getting Alzheimer's disease.

By 2051 the Maori population is expected to reach one million. Thirteen per cent will then be aged over 65 years of age, and the number of Maori with Alzheimer's disease will rise. We need to consider now how best to provide acceptable care to Maori with dementia. Unfortunately, diseases that damage blood vessels — diabetes, high cholesterol and high blood pressure — are common in Maori. And as these disorders increase the likelihood of developing vascular dementia, Maori have a higher incidence of this, and it often occurs at a younger age than does Alzheimer's.

Beliefs and attitudes

In Maori culture health encompasses physical (te taha tinana), spritual (te taha wairua), mental (te taha hinengaro) and family wellbeing (te taha whanau). People are valued for a wider set of characteristics than merely the cognitive or intellectual skills, so someone with dementia may be more accepted by the community.

However, traditionally Maori see life as balance between tapu, that which is sacred or off limits, and noa, that which is relaxed and has no restrictions. Transgression of tapu can result in suffering. Illness, such as dementia, may be seen as the result of such a transgression and thus be regarded as shameful, whakama.

Either acceptance of the person's condition or the shame associated with it may deter people from seeking help. As a result, Maori elders usually come to health services later in the disease, often at a time of crisis.

Assessment

It may be difficult for younger people to acknowledge that a respected older person is becoming forgetful or not coping well. People may cover up and make excuses for the person to avoid facing the issue. While this preserves mana, it may mean that kaumatua and kuia who would benefit from assistance do not get it. Certainly, it may be difficult to respectfully persuade a person to go for an assessment. It may also be difficult to speak frankly about that person's problems, especially in their presence.

Assessment cannot be rushed. If the doctor does not first get to know the person with dementia and their whanau, and gain their confidence, the patient may seem more confused than they usually are. No one need be assessed alone. Whanau should always be welcome, both for support and as a source of information. Hopefully, the assessing staff will remember to ask whether people want a member of the Maori Health Team present. If they do not, family members can ask for this. However, staff of specific cultural services don't always know a great deal about dementia. Some branches of Alzheimer's New Zealand have Maori field workers, who can be supportive at any stage of the disease.

It may take some time for Maori families/whanau to feel at ease with a non-Maori health professional, but they must establish a good relationship before going on to the next stage of assessment. The assessment does not have to be completed in one sitting or within any time limit. Although people may regard the doctor or nurse as an authority figure, it is important that they do not agree to do anything that makes them uncomfortable or that they are not going to be able to keep up. The tests used in assessment, for example, the MMSE, can be humiliating for anyone, especially for someone who is regarded with esteem. Language, education levels and beliefs affect the results of many psychological tests, which are geared for white, middle-class people. A good dementia assessment is holistic and should consider the four cornerstones of wellbeing — physical, spiritual, mental and family. Western medicine needs to incorporate the cultural belief of the patient.

Services

Maori society is diverse. Some Maori are comfortable in mainstream health services; others prefer a specifically Maori programme that includes traditional healing. A few District Health Boards fund traditional healers. Often both types of service can work together. In some areas there are specific Maori day programmes provided.

Many Maori like to have Maori provide care within the mainstream services. However, most of the people employed in old-age health services are non-Maori.

Services such as Meals on Wheels or residential care facilities may not provide the sort of food that some Maori prefer. There are few rest homes or day care facilities specifically for Maori. However, this need has been recognised and some services have been put in place. There are some Maori home care providers.

One Maori man talking about his experience in respite care, said:

> I am very fussy with my food. I like plenty of salt — Pakeha don't put salt in.

> The first time, I enjoyed the food. The second time I couldn't stomach it, so I asked for some hangi — I can eat hangi till the cows come home.[8]

It is important that Maori people using dementia services give feedback to providers so they can adapt the services to suit.

Ongoing care

There is often an assumption that a Maori family will look after their elders, but while whanau may want to do this it can be difficult, especially for urban Maori. Adult children have to work and despite their best intentions may not be able to offer adequate care. A survey in Auckland showed that Maori use rest home care at the same rate as Pakeha.[9]

Participants at hui to discuss this '. . . acknowledged that there is an increasing incidence of kaumatua being separated from their families or whanau due to changing living and working patterns which can leave older people socially isolated'.[10]

A relative caring for a person with dementia fulltime at home can receive the Domestic Purposes Benefit (DPB). Alternatively, a family member can be paid to come in during the day to provide care in the person's home (see chapter 11). Having family provide personal care is often more acceptable to the older person than having a stranger coming in.

Maori traditional healing is more active than just accepting treatment from a health professional. It requires the involvement and faith of the individual and the participation of the family. Herbs, massage, rituals and interpretation of symbols may all be used in this form of healing.

Prayer and blessings (karakia) are important in all aspects of Maori life, including health problems. Karakia may be included in assessment, meetings to decide about treatment and ongoing care, in the final stages of life and after death. Similarly, family involvement, whanau support, is essential at all stages of the journey of the person with dementia.

Hallucinations that occur in dementia may not be regarded as a problem and are sometimes seen as a spiritual gift. Thus, there is no need to treat them unless the person becomes distressed. Even then, medication will not necessarily be the first line of treatment. Various forms of traditional healing may be effective in calming the person or making sense of the experience. Sometimes, people with dementia are venerated because they are released from the shackles of reason and so free to develop their intuitive nature.

Pacific Island peoples

There are many different Pacific cultures. Older people who are recent arrivals in New Zealand will have different needs from people who have been here for decades and are used to the country. Living in New Zealand can be very different from Pacific people's previous lifestyle where they may have been able to live off the land and there is not so much pressure for young people to work long hours in order to support the family. In Pacific communities with a less frenetic lifestyle, older people are freer to do their own thing: to visit the grandchildren when they wish or to walk around. If a person with dementia wanders off, local people know who they are and can return them home. The warmer climate reduces the risk of hypothermia.

In New Zealand, however, older people may speak poor English and have little community support. Often they have to mind the grandchildren while the parents are both out working. If the older person develops dementia and can no longer be safely left in charge, childcare and working arrangements break down. This may increase financial stress. Poverty, overcrowding and breakdown of community support put pressure on families who are trying to cope with a relative with dementia. If they do not have transport or a telephone, it can be difficult to arrange and get to appointments.

Beliefs and attitudes

The Pacific view of health is holistic: mental, physical and spiritual health are all necessary for wellbeing. It is important to understand the person's place within the family and in relation to their ancestors. Many Pacific people believe that any form of disability is a punishment for past sins, not only of the individual, but also of the family. Some churches hold this view also. Mental illness is often seen as being caused by the breaking of custom, resulting in the anger of spiritual forces. This means that people may feel ashamed and not want to admit there is anything wrong with the person with dementia. If they seek help, they will first go to family members, then to community elders or the church before attending a doctor.

Assessment and services

Family members should always attend the assessment with the person. To meet Pacific people's needs, workers have to understand the language, customs, values, attitudes and beliefs involved. Unfortunately, there are few Pacific Island workers employed by public health services for older people, though many District Health Boards have Pacific support units. People can ask for a health worker from their culture to be involved in the assessment and treatment of their family member. Hospitals also provide interpreters. Your local branch of Alzheimer's New Zealand may have a Pacific Island person working with them who can attend the assessment if requested.

Ongoing care

Care at home is preferable to residential care if the family see it as their responsibility to look after older people. Many Pacific Island people hate to have their bodies touched by people who are not family members, so that mainstream home help services and residential care may be unacceptable. However, Needs Assessment and Service Coordination (NASC) may be able to arrange funding to allow a suitable family member to care for the person with dementia. There are now a few rest homes run by and for Pacific Island people and many Pacific Island people work in residential care. It is very comforting for people with dementia to have someone around who speaks their language and appreciates their customs, especially if they have had to go and live in a strange place.

Indian/South Asian

Many people from different parts of the vast Indian subcontinent live in New Zealand. They have arrived in various waves over the years, often via Fiji or Africa, and have adopted New Zealand culture to a greater or lesser degree. Education levels among older people vary immensely. There is no one consistent primary language or religion, and to accommodate this the following comments are very broad.

Beliefs and attitudes

Traditionally there are very strong family links and belonging to the group is very important. Outside the family, with its hierarchical control system, people may feel that they have lost their identity. Often the older women have the task of trying to keep the multi-generational group together. There is not a high level of awareness of dementia in this community and people may not understand why someone is acting in an unusual way.

Stigma is associated with any form of mental illness and this may prevent families from seeking help or mean that the person complains of physical rather than mental symptoms, confusing the picture. Because of the level of stigma, people receiving dementia services need to be absolutely certain of confidentiality. They may not necessarily trust interpreters who could be part of their own community.

Services

There is a range of traditional healers available, even in New Zealand. Religious leaders, astrologers, Ayurvedic practitioners and others may be consulted before turning to Western medicine. Many Indian people are reasonably comfortable with European medicine, and there are many practitioners of Indian sub-continental origin. Women often prefer a female doctor.

Ongoing care

Families still prefer to look after their older people themselves and there are traditional patterns to this. For example, it is the responsibility of the oldest son to care for his mother (actually, the duty often falls to the daughter-in-law). As the younger generations become more Westernised, this pattern is beginning to break down (even in India). It is hard for older people to accept that the family is not going to care for them and that they will have to live in residential care. This can lead to much distress for the older people and their families. If residential care is necessary, clients and families prefer there to be staff of a similar background employed. Older Indian people may struggle with the language and the food. There are some specific support services for them, such as Shanti Niwas in Auckland, which is a charitable trust working with senior citizens of Indian and South Asian origin. See www.shantiniwas.org.nz

Chinese

People of Chinese ethnic origin form a significant part of our population. There is a great deal of diversity in this group: from the descendants of Chinese people who immigrated during the gold rush years, who are now well integrated into New Zealand society, to the many recent immigrants. These immigrants come from a variety of backgrounds so it is not possible to make any assumptions about their culture. Older people who migrated recently to join their children may speak very little English. They can be very isolated, relying on their families (who are often working all day) for support and care should they get ill.

Beliefs and attitudes

Recent Chinese immigrants tend to regard mental illness as shameful and thus may not readily seek treatment if there are signs of dementia in themselves or their families. They may be reluctant to use an interpreter because they fear the person will talk about them to the community. (Professional interpreters are, however, bound by the same rules of confidentiality as other health staff.) As it is acceptable to be physically ill, the person with dementia may express distress by complaining about physical rather than emotional or cognitive symptoms. People who are recent immigrants may have more trust in traditional herbal and other remedies, though often accept Western medicine as well.

Services

Mandarin- and Cantonese-speaking doctors may be able to assess the person and make a diagnosis of dementia more easily than those who have to rely on an interpreter. There are many GPs who speak one of these languages and there are often speakers of Chinese dialects in the hospital services.

Ongoing care

Because communication is a problem for anyone with dementia, it is helpful to have people who speak the person's first language caring for them. Some rest homes provide care for Chinese people, with Cantonese- and Mandarin-speaking staff. There are some specific day programmes available for Chinese elders in Auckland. As well as language, there are issues around religion, customs, food and activities that need to be addressed if the person is in permanent residential care. The cultural habits of a lifetime need to be maintained, even when the person has dementia, in order to appreciate that person as a person.

In summary

People with dementia need to have their identity affirmed. As the disease progresses, other people have the important task of helping them to maintain meaning, spirituality and personhood.

References

[1] Frankl, Victor, *Man's Search for Meaning,* Washington Square Press, New York, 1984.

[2] Bellah, Robert N., *Habits of the Heart: Individualism and commitment in American life*, with Richard Madeson, William M. Sullivan, Ann Swider, Steven M. Tipton, University of California Press, Berkeley, 1985, pp. 246–7.

[3] Kitwood, Tom, *Dementia Reconsidered: The person comes first*, Open University Press, Buckingham, 1997.

[4] Boden, Christine, *Who Will I Be When I Die?*, HarperCollins, Sydney, 1997.

[5] MacKinley, Elizabeth, *The Spiritual Dimension of Ageing*, Jessica Kingsley Publishers, London, 2001.

[6] Kitwood, Tom, *Dementia Reconsidered*, 1997.

[7] 'The Social Report', 2010, http://socialreport.msd.govt.nz/health/life-expectancy.html, and Koopman-Boyden, Peggy, 'The Story: Older people', Te Ara — The Encyclopedia of

New Zealand, http://www.teara.govt.nz/en/older-people/1, licensed by Manatū Taonga for re-use under the Creative Commons Attribution-NonCommercial 3.0 New Zealand Licence. Both websites accessed on 3 November 2012.

8 'Mental Health Services for Older People', Northern Regional Service Plan, consultation document, 2000.

9 Richmond, D., Baskett, J., Bonita, R. et al. *Care for Older People in New Zealand: A report to the National Advisory Committee on Core Health and Disability Support Services*. Published by National Advisory Committee on Core Health and Disability Services, Wellington, 1995.

10 Ministry of Health, *The Health and Wellbeing of Older People and Kaumatua: The public health issues*, Wellington, 1997.

Chapter 17
Legal and ethical issues

Atawhai Tia o Matua
Whakanuia o Tupuna
Whakahonore Tia o Ratou
Matauranga

Cherish your parents
Salute your elders
Honour their wisdom

PROVERB

Legal issues arise at some point for most people during the course of their dementia. The most common question is, 'Who will make decisions for me when I am no longer able to?'

The laws most relevant to people with dementia are as follows:

- The Protection of Personal and Property Rights Act (1988)
- The Mental Health Act (1992)
- The Human Rights Act, which forbids discrimination against people on grounds of age or disability
- The Health and Disability Commissioner Act, if the person with dementia is not happy with their treatment from the health or aged care services
- The Privacy Act, which can cause problems if people don't understand it.

In this chapter I also discuss guidelines for driving, making a will and ways of dealing with elder abuse.

The Protection of Personal and Property Rights Act

In its own words the Protection of Personal and Property Rights Act (PPPR Act) 'provides for the protection and promotion of the personal and property rights of persons who are not fully able to manage their own affairs'.

Personal rights are about deciding where someone lives, and what medical treatment and support they have. Property rights are about people's financial arrangements, their property (such as a house or shares) and who will manage them when the owner can no longer do so. People who cannot make decisions are said to 'lack capacity' (or 'be lacking competence'). The PPPR Act encourages people who lack capacity to have as much say as possible in what happens to them, but as well, they need to be protected from harm. Sometimes this is a difficult balance.

Parts of the PPPR Act

There are basically four parts to the Act: personal orders, welfare guardians, property managers and enduring power of attorney.

Personal Orders

A judge (usually in the Family Court) can order that a person:

- Undergo treatment; for example, have an operation, take medication, receive home care
- Live in a particular place; for example, go to a rest home even if the person objects, be brought back there if he or she has left, live in a 'secure' environment such as a dementia unit
- Be admitted to hospital (but not a psychiatric ward); for example, if they are physically ill, but won't go or can't decide to go.

Welfare guardian

The court appoints a person, the welfare guardian, to make decisions about 'welfare', that is, personal and health decisions such as those listed above. A welfare guardian is appointed if the person is totally lacking capacity, i.e. cannot make any decisions either in a particular area (for example, where to live) or in any area at all. The welfare guardian has the power to make decisions in the aspects of care where the person is incapable. Usually a family member is appointed as the welfare guardian. If there is no one available to act as a welfare guardian, organisations such as Age Concern may have a volunteer willing to take on this role, but it is often difficult to find someone to do this responsible job. When families cannot agree on who should be the welfare guardian, then the court has to decide who will be the best person. The welfare guardian must try to involve the person with dementia in the decision-making process.

Property manager

If someone who lacks capacity has property worth more than $10,000, a property manager can be appointed by the court to look after the person's financial affairs. The property manager can pay bills (including rest home or hospital fees), buy or sell property or shares and run a business. The property manager can also make changes to the person's will if they think it no longer reflects the person's intentions. Often the property manager is a family member, but trusts, such as the Public Trust or the Guardian Trust, can also provide this service for a fee. Property managers have to report annually to the court to show that they are managing the person's property appropriately. If they are not sure what to do in a certain situation they can apply to the court for advice.

Enduring Power of Attorney (EPOA)

While a person still has capacity he or she can appoint someone (an 'attorney') to manage their affairs — welfare or property or both. (Despite the legal-sounding name, an attorney does not have to be a lawyer.) Often people appoint one person to make decisions about welfare (a daughter?) and another to manage property (a son?). When writing an EPOA, people can be as specific or as broad as they like. For example, they could appoint someone to make all welfare decisions or just to decide about residential care. The attorney takes over the management of the person's affairs when the person is unable to do so, i.e. when they become 'incapacitated'. However, if someone who still has capacity would like their property managed by the attorney, then they can hand over that power whenever they want.

If:

(1) the person's property management will be complicated or
(2) there is friction in the family or
(3) there is a possibility of a conflict of interest between the person with dementia and the attorney,

it may be better to get a property manager appointed so that the accounts are audited annually through the courts.

By making an EPOA people with dementia can have their say about what happens in the future, when they might be unable to express their wishes. This means that the stress and cost of going to court to appoint a welfare guardian or property manager later can usually be avoided. Only one person can be EPOA for welfare, but more than one person or a trustee company (e.g., The Public Trust) can be EPOA for property.

Using the PPPR Act

Enduring Power of Attorney

Previously people could just download the forms or write their own EPOA papers. However, because there have been instances of abuse, e.g., getting someone to sign a form that they didn't understand or pressuring them to do it, an EPOA must now be made with a lawyer. The lawyer has to be quite certain that the person appointing the attorney understands what they are doing. This law change makes it less likely that abuse will occur, however it has meant that some people don't appoint an EPOA because of legal costs.

Alzheimer's New Zealand, Age Concern or a Citizens Advice Bureau can assist people to make an EPOA. A useful link is www.ageconcern.org.nz/money/planning/enduring-power-attorney

When the person with dementia becomes unable to manage their affairs, then the EPOA is activated. The law now requires that a doctor writes a letter to confirm that the person lacks capacity. This then allows the EPOA to take over decision-making *but* they must still consult as much as possible with the person with dementia.

Other orders

The making of personal orders and the appointment of a welfare guardian or property manager must be done through the court, so it is best to involve a lawyer. However, it is possible for any concerned person to make an application. The appropriate forms can be obtained from the Family Court or downloaded from www.courts.govt.nz/family/pppr. However, if it has become necessary to appoint a welfare guardian or property manager, it is likely that the person with dementia will already have a social worker who can direct the process.

Once the application forms are filled out and the medical report on capacity completed, the papers are filed at the Family Court. The court appoints a lawyer (or counsel) on behalf of the person with dementia, who investigates the best options for the person and then makes recommendations to the court. This is done in a pre-hearing conference, with the person with dementia, their social worker, family and any other relevant parties present. If it would be pointless or distressing for the person with dementia to attend, then they are excused. The court may then request further information, such as medical reports, or it might make the order. The Family Court, while reasonably formal, is not particularly scary, and judges try to make sure everyone understands what is happening.

Once the order is made

If a personal order is made, the person with dementia will be told to accept treatment, live in a rest home or do whatever else the order says. Once appointed, a welfare guardian has to organise whatever needs to be done; for example, get home help or take the person to a care facility. Usually, the person with dementia will go along with what a court has ordered or what they are told they must do by the welfare guardian. It is not clear whether the Act allows the welfare guardian to forcibly take the person into care, but most guardians manage to get around the problem in other ways if the person with dementia objects. When appointed, the property manager can officially take control of the person's financial affairs.

Ex parte order

The court process can take a long time. If the situation is urgent, then the judge can make an order (for example, that the person have medical attention or be admitted to care) after reviewing the papers that have been filled out, but without seeing the person. This is called an ex parte order and can be requested by submitting another form that explains why the situation is urgent. A social worker or medical team is likely to be involved and would help decide when to ask for an ex parte order.

Duration of an order

Once in place, the order lasts three years at most, though the judge may ask for an earlier review. The order lapses after three years if someone does not ask for it to be renewed.

Mismanagement issues

If the person appointed as welfare guardian or property manager appears not to be doing the job properly, anyone can apply to the court for a review.

Testing for capacity

People do not lack capacity just because they have been diagnosed with dementia. In fact, the law states:

> For the purposes of this part of the Act, every person shall be presumed, until the contrary is proved, to have the capacity . . . to understand the nature and to foresee the consequences of decisions in respect of matters.

That is, the person is assumed to be able to make decisions unless it is proven that they cannot.

Usually it is a doctor (occasionally a psychologist) who writes a report to say whether or not a person has the capacity to make decisions. There is no formal or standard way to do a capacity assessment. It depends on what the assessment is for. For example, if someone is being assessed to see if they are capable of appointing someone to be an EPOA, then that person will need to understand what an EPOA is, who might be appointed and why, when it will come into action and that it can be changed if they so choose. The person's decision should also be in line with previous thinking, for example, a recent acquaintance should not be appointed in preference to a daughter who has been caring for the person for years. If the assessment is to see whether a person needs a property manager, then it will focus more on the person's understanding of what their assets, income and outgoings are and also the person's ability to calculate, read bank statements and write cheques.

To complicate matters, people may be only partly (rather than wholly) incapacitated, meaning that they can make decisions about some things and not others. A man who has had a stroke might not be able to calculate or write cheques, but could still have some say in the overall running of his business and be able to make his own decisions about welfare matters. Capacity can also vary over time. People with dementia have good times and bad times during the day and their capacity may fluctuate depending on their physical or emotional state. They may be able to make reasonable decisions on good days.

> *When I first visited Mrs N., she had a chest infection and was very confused. She was not able to make coherent statements about anything. When I came back a week later, she was quite clear she wanted to appoint her daughter as an EPOA and was able to give good reasons for doing so. I believed she had the capacity to appoint an attorney.*

As dementia progresses, however, capacity reduces.

Advance directives, advance care plans and living wills

Advance directives and living wills are instructions left for a person to make decisions, usually about end-of-life care (see chapter 14). They could be included with an EPOA, so that the attorney can take into account what the person with dementia would have wanted in the way of medical treatment.

There is also provision under the Health and Disability Commissioner Act to make an advance directive. Making an advance directive is quite complicated and rarely done. However, this is a good time to have a discussion about the sort of things that you think will be important to you in future and write them down. See www.advancecareplanning.org.nz to get some ideas.

Making or changing a will

People in the early stages of dementia would be wise to update or make a will if they haven't already done so. Even at this stage — and definitely later — it is worth getting a medical certificate to say the person with dementia is competent to make or change a will, that is, that the person has testamentary capacity. This can save expensive court battles after death in which people argue over whether or not the person with dementia really understood what he or she was doing.

To make a will a person needs to:

- Know what a will is
- Know that it takes force after their death
- Know the extent of his or her assets and liabilities; i.e. what he or she owns and has in the bank, or owes
- Know who might have a claim on the assets; i.e. family members who could expect to benefit from the will (and be able to justify leaving these people out if that is what he or she wants)
- Not be coerced; i.e. under pressure to make changes or favour a particular person.

Note that if a person changes a will after a diagnosis of dementia, the onus is on them to prove that they are competent. They are not presumed to 'have capacity', as in the PPPR Act. There are several local websites with information about making a will, for example, see www.consumer.org.nz/reports/wills

Mental Health Act

The Mental Health (Compulsory Assessment and Treatment) Act (1992) (MHA) defines the circumstances in which people suffering from mental disorder may be treated without their consent. The Act is intended to protect their rights.

While the Act is usually invoked to treat people with acute mental disorders, it can be applied to dementia in situations where the person's condition places them in danger and a rapid response is required. Usually, the person needs admission to a psychiatric ward for their own safety or that of others. Under the MHA this can happen if their 'abnormal state of mind . . . poses a serious danger to the health or safety of that person or of others' or 'seriously diminishes the capacity of that person to take care of himself or herself'.

The most common situations in which the MHA is used are:

- When a person becomes acutely confused and puts themselves or others in danger, i.e. develops delirium on top of the dementia
- When someone with dementia develops delusions or hallucinations and won't accept help or threatens others
- When a person who is chronically at risk (for example, from self-neglect or unsafe behaviours) refuses assessment or assistance because they believe there is nothing wrong.

Family will almost always be involved in the decision to use the MHA and they should be kept informed of the process along the way. If family or friends believe that the person with dementia is in imminent danger, they can contact the local Mental Health Crisis service. If the Crisis Service decides that the person should be placed under the MHA, then a 'duly authorised officer' (usually a psychiatric nurse) makes the arrangements for assessment. Two doctors, one of whom must be a psychiatrist, interview the patient and decide whether the use of the MHA is justified. Although the Act allows for compulsory treatment in the community, the situation is usually so unstable that the person needs to be admitted to a mental health ward.

It can be difficult getting a person in this state to hospital. However, once they are told they must be admitted, they will often go along with it. If the police have to be involved the sight of a few blue uniforms can be enough to persuade someone to go quietly. In my experience the police are very good with older and confused people, dealing with them with just the right mixture of kindness and firmness. This can be very traumatic for all concerned, leaving people wondering if they have done the right thing. Usually, however, it is the only option and the person settles once they are in the ward.

How the Mental Health Act works

The Act allows for up to 19 days to assess and treat the person with dementia. By this time, things have usually settled down sufficiently for the person to be discharged or agree to stay in hospital. If not, the psychiatrist applies for a Compulsory Treatment Order. The patient, family and treating doctors then appear at a Family Court hearing (usually held at the hospital) to argue for more time to treat the patient. A lawyer, provided through Legal Aid, is appointed to represent the patient. It is very helpful to have the family attend the hearing to put their views forward on the best plan of management. The patient will eventually be discharged from the hospital, possibly still under the MHA or the PPPR Act, if this seems more suitable. The person can be removed from the MHA at any time the doctor thinks fit. If they stay under the MHA they are reviewed and a report sent to the court every three months. If the family, or the patient, object to the MHA being used they can ask for a judge's review under Section 16 of the Act.

Mr L. refused to see a doctor about his failing memory. He denied that there was anything wrong with him, although his wife had gradually taken over more and more of his care. He became increasingly irritable and threatened but never hit Mrs L. One night he became acutely confused. He was hallucinating and tried to climb out the window of his house. His wife could not get near him because he lashed out, apparently unaware of who she was.

He was put under the MHA as he had a 'disorder of cognition and perceptions', which endangered his wife and made him unable to care for himself. He was taken to hospital and treated, although he could not agree to this.

During the initial five-day period of assessment he was found to have a bladder infection that made him delirious. Once this was treated he became more amenable and agreed to stay in the ward while his dementia was investigated, so he was discharged from the MHA. He returned home to the care of his wife, who made an application to be his welfare guardian under the PPPR Act.

Health and Disability Commissioner Act

The Health and Disability Commissioner Act (HDC) protects the rights of people using health or disability services. People with complaints about the care received and who have not made progress through a direct approach to the health care provider (or are reluctant to pursue this) can talk to their local HDC advocate. The advocate listens to concerns, helps clarify the issues, gives information about rights, provides options to resolve the issue and supports the person or family making a complaint. The advocate tries to sort things out informally before going on to a full investigation. The formal investigations tend to take months rather than days or weeks.

Consumers of health and disability services have the following rights:

1. To be treated with respect
2. To freedom from discrimination, coercion, harassment and exploitation
3. To dignity and independence
4. To services of an appropriate standard
5. To effective communication
6. To be fully informed
7. To make an informed choice and give informed consent
8. To support (i.e. to have someone of their choice present while receiving a health or disability service)
9. To decline involvement in teaching and training
10. To complain.

Health providers are obliged to display information on how to make a complaint. The HDC national number is 0800 112 233 and the website is www.hdc.org.nz/complaints/

Privacy Act

The Privacy Act requires that health care staff must not disclose personal information about patients without their permission. If the person with dementia lacks the capacity to decide whether to release information then their guardian or next of kin decides who is told about the person's condition.

Most people with dementia agree that their close family members should know about their condition and can give permission for the doctor to share information with them. However, sometimes the person with dementia does not want anyone told and cannot be persuaded otherwise. If they are competent to make that decision, staff have to respect it. Only if the person's situation is dangerous (to themselves or others) can they break this privacy. This is a medical decision and may need to be justified later if the person complains.

Information that is necessary for ongoing care can be shared with other health professionals. If employers or insurance companies want medical information this can only be supplied with the person's (preferably written) permission. The Privacy Act also allows people (or their legal guardians) to see the information gathered about them and correct it if necessary.

The Human Rights Act

The Act prevents discrimination against people with a disability (including dementia). A person does not have to leave their job or change their accommodation just because they have been diagnosed with dementia.

Some retirement villages object to having people with dementia living in them as they may 'annoy other residents' or 'reduce the tone of the place'. The management might put pressure on them to move out. This is hurtful, especially if the person has been there a long time. It is also discriminatory and probably contravenes the Human Rights Act.

Driving

It is sometimes difficult to stop someone driving when they are no longer safe. Driving is a sign of independence and freedom. People often feel trapped and useless if they cannot drive. If a partner is dependent on the person with dementia for transport they may be reluctant to acknowledge that driving is a problem.

The mechanics of driving (such as when to change gears) stays with people for a long time. They can drive 'on automatic', hardly aware of where they are, but there are many times when they need to be alert and make snap judgements depending on the conditions.

The problems with driving may depend on what sort of dementia the person has. The list that follows will apply to some people with dementia at some time:

- Getting lost
- Forgetting the road rules
- Slowness of response
- Trouble telling right from left
- Poor coordination
- Loss of distance perception and judgement of speed
- 'Over-the-top' emotional reactions to minor driving incidents
- Poor judgement and decision-making
- Visual changes after a stroke
- Epileptic fits or other causes of loss of consciousness
- Other physical conditions
- Medication affecting alertness.

In the early stages, people with dementia do not necessarily have to stop driving, but others should let them know if they are concerned. Often people limit their driving to the local area during quiet times of day and may be safe enough doing this for a while. If family or friends are frightened when being driven by the person with dementia, if the car is getting dented from numerous minor accidents or if the person has trouble driving along familiar routes, alarm bells should be sounded. Despite a lot of recent research there is no one way to decide when driving should stop. The most consistent sign is that you are frightened of driving with them. Put this question 'Would you let your grandchildren drive with them?' If the answer is 'No', then follow these steps.

Steps to stop someone driving

Most people with dementia recognise when they are having trouble driving and stop of their own volition. However, there are times when others need to intervene. Here are some suggestions on how to do this:

1. Express your concerns and ask the person to stop driving. Offer to do the driving yourself if you can. Suggest alternative means of transport — the train, bus or taxi. Age Concern or Alzheimer's New Zealand can provide the person with dementia with half-price taxi vouchers. 'Driving Miss Daisy' is a service specially set up for older or disabled people.
2. If the person refuses to listen, get a person in authority such as a respected family member, a doctor or a religious leader to talk to the person.
3. If the person is nearly due for a medical check-up for their driving licence, go with them to report on the driving difficulties or phone the doctor beforehand with your concerns. The doctor can bear your information in mind during the medical check-up: the person may then fail and lose their licence.
4. At 75 years a doctor's certificate is required for a licence. After the age of 80, two yearly medical certificates are required and if the doctor recommends it, an on-road safety test (total cost, with licence, $60.50). The licence may then not be renewed; this often causes a major falling out between doctor and patient, so some GPs prefer to refer to a specialist to make decisions about driving.
5. Have the person referred by their GP to a Driving Assessment Service. In some places this is part of the DHB occupational therapy service and is free. In other areas a private occupational therapist does the testing. (It can cost at least $350 for the test.) These services can advise the person to stop driving or recommend adaptations to the car or limitations to the extent of driving. The AA will do a less comprehensive on-road test for about $85 but these people do not have any clinical training.

Even if their licence is revoked, some people still keep on driving. (Either they have forgotten they don't have a licence or they never took much notice of the rules anyway.) More drastic action is then required.

1. Get the local community constable to talk to the person. A visit from the police can sometimes be persuasive.
2. Hide the keys.
3. Put the car in a different place where it is hard for the person to find it.
4. Disable the car. Remove the spark plugs, take out the battery or otherwise prevent it from starting.
5. Sell the car (perhaps having first arranged for it to 'break down', so it needs to be taken to the garage).

Stopping someone driving is a hard thing to do, but it is better than them killing themselves or someone else.

Elder abuse

Estimates suggest that 2 to 5 per cent of older people suffer from abuse. In New Zealand this works out at between 8000 and 21,000 people. It is most commonly women who are abused. They may be living alone (37 per cent), with family (44 per cent) or in residential care (19 per cent). Many of the victims will have dementia, although the exact numbers are unknown. Most abusers are members of the victim's family: about 25 per cent are the person's main carer.

Types of elder abuse

Psychological abuse (approximately 37 per cent). This is any behaviour that threatens, frightens, humiliates or intimidates the older person. The abuser might belittle, yell at or threaten to stop looking after a dependent person.

Financial/material abuse (approximately 30 per cent). This means that someone uses the older person's money or property illegally or improperly. An example might be of people talking the person with dementia into selling them the house for a very low price.

Physical abuse (approximately 13 per cent). The abuser physically hurts the older person perhaps by slapping or pushing them. Tying a person in a chair or overusing medication could be forms of physical abuse.

Active and passive neglect (approximately 12 per cent). This is the failure of the caregiver to provide necessary food, shelter, clothing or medical care. This might be deliberate (active neglect) or for other reasons, such as ignorance, illness or lack of resources (passive neglect).

Sexual abuse (approximately 2 per cent). This includes forcing sexual activity on someone who doesn't want it or who is unable to consent.

Signs of elder abuse

Older people often have very fragile skin that bruises easily, and they are prone to falls, so injuries can occur even with gentle handling and are not necessarily the result of abuse. People with dementia can forget where they left their money and believe that someone has stolen it or they may be unreasonably suspicious of a carer's motives.

Nevertheless, concerns are raised if the person:

- seems afraid of someone
- avoids answering questions about care
- stays awake at night
- becomes depressed or withdrawn
- has recurrent injuries, especially ones that look as if they could be caused by abuse
- is over-sedated
- recoils from being touched
- has injuries in the genital area or fears being taken to the toilet
- is poorly nourished or clothed, has poor hygiene or is cold
- is left alone for long periods without stimulation or visitors
- doesn't use glasses, hearing aids, dentures or take medication as directed
- has bills unpaid when someone is meant to be doing this
- has money (including savings) or possessions disappear
- sells property but is confused about the reasons for its sale.

The abuser may:

- not want the older person to be seen alone and may limit visitors
- treat the older person like a child, threaten, bully or blame them for behaviour which is the result of dementia (such as wandering or incontinence)
- refuse to seek medical treatment for the person or go to different doctors at different times
- be evasive, make excuses or be hostile towards someone who tries to help
- seem very controlling.

There are many reasons for elder abuse. Often it is a complex interaction between old family relationship patterns, caregiver stress and the symptoms of the person with dementia. The carer may feel trapped in the role and not know about other services that would relieve their burden. Alternatively, unscrupulous people may exploit a confused older person for their assets.

What to do?

If you think someone you know is being abused or neglected, you can talk to Elder Abuse Services. These are established throughout the country, and run by Age Concern or Presbyterian Support Services. The community constable, victim support services run by the police or your local Citizens Advice Bureau may be able to help. Phone numbers are in the local phone directory. There are specific services for Maori in some areas. For your local elder abuse service, see www.ageconcern.org.nz/safety/elder-abuse/elder-abuse-and-neglect-prevention-service

Other ethical issues

In the course of the book I have considered ethical issues at the point they seemed most relevant. There are still areas that I haven't addressed, such as what to do if someone is being exploited financially, but appears happy with the exploitative relationship (perhaps because they fear being left alone). I have not touched on how much of society's resources we should put into dementia care. Does the age and condition of people with dementia determine the level of care they will receive? I have also not considered questions about research. Can people with dementia take part in research if they are unable to give informed consent? Should someone else be able to consent on their behalf? If no research is done because people cannot give consent, future people with dementia will miss out on the advances of science.

There is rarely an obvious right answer (it wouldn't be an ethical dilemma if there was). The person with dementia, in the centre of the dilemma, must always be recognised as a person who deserves respect. (See selected reading list for books of interest in this field.)

In summary

We hope that people with dementia will be treated as people with the same rights as everyone else. However, there will always be occasions when they require the protection of the law to ensure that these rights are respected.

Conclusion

Do not go gentle into that good night,
Old age should burn and rave at close of day;
Rage, rage against the dying of the light.
DYLAN THOMAS

It never ceases to amaze me how those closely involved in the care and support of people with dementia can continue to do the right thing by those who cannot speak for themselves. I'm not just thinking of family members and caregivers in rest homes and hospitals, but also those who take on responsibilities such as being a welfare guardian, or work as volunteers to advocate for and assist people with dementia. Care and respect for people with dementia in New Zealand has greatly improved over the last few decades but, as always, there is much more to be done.

We can learn by listening to people with dementia, allowing them to describe their experience and needs. From them we can come to value attributes other than cognitive ability and economic productivity.

We need to improve home care services and develop more innovative and flexible ways to deliver them. We should recognise family caregivers by providing adequate assistance, respite care and emotional support. As a community we need to acknowledge the important job they do. We need to pay professional caregivers well, give excellent training and supervision, and recognise their very valuable contribution.

The role of rest homes and private hospitals is continuing to evolve. There is an increasing adoption of person-centred care and a recognition of individual needs. We should consider alternative types of sheltered accommodation when care in the person's own home is impossible: group homes, sheltered housing, serviced apartments. We must continue to look outside the rest home square. Recently we have formed a National Dementia Cooperative (http://ndc.hiirc.org.nz) that aims to coordinate New Zealand's efforts to improve dementia recognition and care in the areas on research, advocacy, workforce development, informal caregivers, information sharing and dementia care pathways.

We must understand that having dementia does not mean that the people with it cease to be human beings; the rights of such vulnerable people must be protected. It is vitally important that we recognise that it is still possible for people to live well with dementia and must continue to work so this is a reality. Whatever we, who have 'temporarily able brains', do for people with dementia now, might improve our own situation in the future.

I hope this book has gone a little way to addressing some of the fears and prejudices we have about dementia so that we can be more understanding and compassionate towards these people and those who care for them.

> He aha te mea tino nui: he tangata, he tangata, he tangata.
> What is the most important thing in life? It is people; it is people; it is people.

Glossary

Acetylcholine: a neurotransmitter important in memory and other areas. Low levels in most dementias

Acetylcholinesterase: an enzyme (chemical) that breaks down acetylcholine

Acetylcholinesterase inhibitor: a drug that stops acetylcholinesterase from working (and hence raises the level of acetylcholine)

Agnosia: inability to recognise things

Alzheimer's disease: the most common form of dementia

Amygdala: an area of the brain important for memory

Amyloid: a protein laid down in the brain and body in response to injury

Anti-anxiety medication: also called minor tranquillisers. Pills used to calm down anxious people, most often benzodiazepines

Anticholinergic drugs: medications with many uses that can cause or worsen confusion

Anticonvulsants: drugs to stop fits or seizures

Antidepressants: drugs used to treat the mental illness depression. Also helpful for anxiety and some symptoms of frontotemporal dementia, e.g., citalopram, paroxetine

Antioxidants: drugs that counteract damaging free radicals

Antipsychotics: medication to treat psychotic symptoms such as delusions and hallucinations. Also used to calm people. Sometimes called 'major tranquillisers', e.g., haloperidol, quetiapine

Anxiety: worry. Also a mental illness where worrying has become chronic and out of proportion

Aphasia: language difficulties, trouble finding the name for things

Apraxia: not being able to perform movements or tasks because of brain damage despite having the physical ability to do so

Arteriosclerosis: damage caused to blood vessels making them narrow, irregular, rough and stiff

Artery: a blood vessel taking blood away from the heart towards limbs and vital organs such as the brain. They can contract and expand to keep blood pressure at suitable levels. They can be damaged by arteriosclerosis

Atrial fibrillation: a heart beat irregularity in which blood clots can form in a part of the heart. Later these clots may break off, travel to the brain and cause a stroke

Butyrlcholine: neurotransmitter

Butyrlcholinesterase: an enzyme that breaks down butyrylcholine

Butyrylcholinesterase inhibitor: a drug that stops butyrylcholinesterase from working

CAT scan: computerised axial tomography scan

Cerebrovascular accident: the loss of blood supply to an area of the brain and the outcome of this. Usually caused by a blood clot in a major artery or bleeding into the brain (haemorrhage)

Cholesterol: a fat in the blood. Long term, high levels cause damage to blood vessels

Cognition: a whole range of thinking: includes remembering, reasoning, making decisions, recognising things, applying past experience

Cognition-enhancing drugs: any medications that improve cognition

Cognitive: to do with cognition

Computerised axial tomography scan (CAT scan): a method of X-raying fine slices of the brain to build up a three-dimensional picture of the brain

Cortex: the top part of the brain (where cognition occurs)

CT scan: computerised axial tomography scan

CVA: cerebrovascular accident (stroke)

Delirium/delirious: a state of acute mental confusion, usually caused by physical illness

Delusions: false beliefs that the person cannot be talked out of

Depression: used here as the name of a mental illness (rather than just an unhappy state)

Depth perception: the ability to judge how far away things are and whether one thing is in front of or behind another

Dopamine: a neurotransmitter, low in Parkinson's disease

Down's Syndrome (also known as Down Syndrome): a common form of congenital intellectual disability caused by an abnormal chromosome

Electrolytes: chemicals in the blood, regulated by the kidney

Enduring Power of Attorney or EPOA (also abbreviated to EPA): a person appointed to look after someone's affairs should that person become incapable of doing so himself or herself

Executive function: planning, organising, doing things in order, making judgements, thinking

Free radical: a form of oxygen that damages tissue, including brain tissue, and that also may be responsible for ageing

Frontotemporal dementias: a group of brain diseases affecting the frontal and temporal lobes of the brain

Geriatrician: a physician specialising in the illnesses of old age

Hallucinations: perceiving something that is not there: *visual hallucinations*: seeing things that are not there; *auditory hallucinations*: hearing something when there is no external sound; *tactile hallucinations*: feeling as if touched when there is nothing to touch the person; *olfactory hallucinations*: smelling something when there is no odour; *gustatory hallucinations*: tasting something when there is nothing to taste; *somatic hallucinations*: feeling that something is going on in the body

Hippocampus: an area of the brain thought to be important in memory

Homeopathy: a system of alternative medicine where very small amounts of remedies are used

Huntington's disease: an inherited illness that causes abnormal movements and often dementia

Hydrocephalus: increased fluid around the brain, sometimes with increased pressure on the brain

Hyperintensities: bright areas on an MRI scan of the brain, often where there is poor blood supply

Hyperlipidaemia: high levels of fat in the blood

Hypertension: high blood pressure (causes blood vessel damage)

Hypnotics: pills used to help people get to sleep

Hypoglycaemia: low blood sugar, can starve brain

Hypotension: low blood pressure (can mean not enough blood gets to the brain)

Incidence: the number of new cases (usually of a disease) occurring over a certain period of time, e.g., six new cases a year

Incontinence: loss of control of bladder (urinary incontinence) or bowel (faecal incontinence)

Inhibitions: psychological controls that determine the way we behave, speak and express emotions. Sometimes lost in dementia

Intellectual disability: people with a low intelligence and some difficulties functioning in the world without assistance. Previously called intellectual handicap. In the UK called 'learning disability'

Informant Questionnaire on Cognitive Decline in the Elderly (IQCODE): a 16 or 26 question test measuring cognitive decline

Ischaemia/ischaemic: damage done because of a lack of blood supply

Labile/lability: widely fluctuating emotional responses which are not always appropriate
Lacunae: fluid-filled holes in the brain, often the result of previous small strokes
Language abilities: not just talking, but understanding what is said, regulating one's own speech, reading and writing
Lewy: a scientist studying the brain in the early 20th century
Lewy bodies: objects seen under the microscope in the brains of people with Parkinson's disease and Lewy body dementia
Lewy body dementia: a recently recognised form of dementia which has symptoms like Parkinson's disease
Magnetic resonance imaging: a way of X-raying the brain to get a clearer picture than a CT scan. Especially useful for vascular problems
Malignant social psychology: a way of dealing with people with dementia which makes their disabilities worse
Mental Status Questionnaire (MSQ): a 10-question test for cognitive function
Mini Mental Status Examination (MMSE): a 30-question test for cognitive function (use is decreasing because of copyright issues)
Mixed dementia: dementia caused by both Alzheimer's disease and vascular dementia
Montreal Cognitive Assessment (MOCA): a 30 question test for cognitive function
MRI: magnetic resonance imaging
Nervous system: the brain, spinal cord and peripheral nerves
Neurologist: a specialist doctor trained and experienced in diseases of the nervous system
Neuropsychological testing: extensive tests carried out by psychologists or specialist neuropsychologists to check out brain function
Neurotransmitters: brain chemicals carrying messages between nerve cells (e.g., acetylcholine, butyrlcholine and dopamine)
Orientation: knowing where you are in time and place. Usually tested by asking a person the date and their address
Paranoia: unfounded suspicion that others want to harm the person in some way
Parkinson's disease: a progressive neurological disease. The person develops stiffness, shaking, slowness, shuffling, other physical symptoms and often dementia
Perception: something that is seen, heard, felt, tasted, smelt, something detected by the senses
Personality: the way a person habitually views the world and reacts to events and other people

Person-centred care: a method of caring for people with dementia which puts the person at the centre and tries to understand what is happening for the person
Personhood: the unique person who is still present despite having dementia
Pharmac: government agency that decides which medications will be funded by the government
Physiotherapist: a health professional trained to keep people mobile, also to help with breathing
Pick bodies: microscopic bodies seen inside brain cells affected with Pick's disease
Plaques: amyloid protein laid down in patches in the brain in Alzheimer's disease and to a lesser extent in the other dementias and in normal, ageing brains
Prevalence: the number of cases of something, usually a disease in a community, at any one time, e.g., 20 cases in this area (also see Incidence)
Psychiatrist: a specialist doctor trained in diagnosing and treating mental illness
Psychogeriatrician: a psychiatrist working with older people
Psychologists: people who study and treat people by psychological methods
Psychology: the study of human emotions, cognition and behaviour
Psychotherapy: talking therapy with a trained person to help overcome mental health or emotional problems
Recall: bringing back into awareness something that is in one's memory
Registration: taking in information
Rementing: regaining skills as the result of good person-centred care
Retrieval: finding and bringing back a memory, another word for recall in this book
Sentient: conscious or aware
Shadowing: following a person very closely, not letting them out of sight
Side effects: drug effects that are not the main effect. They may be helpful or cause problems
Spatial awareness: knowing where our bodies are in space, and the things around us in relation to ourselves and other objects
Statins: drugs to reduce the level of unhealthy blood lipids (fats) such as cholesterol
Storage: the keeping of a memory (somewhere in the brain)
Stroke: what happens to a person when the blood supply to part of the brain is lost, often evident as loss of consciousness, weakness of one side of the body, slurring or loss of speech. Also known as a cerebrovascular accident or CVA
Sub-cortex (sub-cortical): the lower part of the brain, important for maintaining life, e.g., breathing, consciousness, not involved in thinking
Sundowning: a pattern of getting agitated and restless in the late afternoon

Tangles: dying nerve tissue in the brains of people with Alzheimer's disease and the other dementias and normal older brains to a lesser extent

Tau: an abnormal protein in the brains of people with Alzheimer's disease and some other dementias

Thyroid: a gland in the neck which can cause problems if over- or underactive. Thyroid function blood tests can check for this

Trailing: following someone around very closely

Tranquillisers: drugs used to calm people

Ubiquitin: abnormal protein in the brains of people with dementia

Vascular: to do with blood vessels

Vascular dementia: a form of dementia caused by lack of blood supply to the brain

Withdrawal: stopping being involved in previous relationships or activities

Useful contacts

General

Alzheimer's New Zealand
National Office Ph: 0800 004 001 or 04 387 8264
Fax: 04 387 9682
nationaloffice@alzheimers.org.nz
www.alzheimers.org.nz
Education and support for people affected by all forms of dementia

National Dementia Cooperative
ndc.hiirc.org.nz
Collaboration of individuals and organisations interested in dementia in New Zealand

Elder Net
Ph: 03 388 1204
Fax: 03 388 1271
www.eldernet.co.nz
team@eldernet.co.nz
Information for older people including community groups, home services, retirement villages, residential/rest home care and private hospitals

Age Concern New Zealand
National Office Ph: 04 801 9338
Fax: 04 801 9336
www.ageconcern.org.nz
national.office@ageconcern.org.nz
Plus there is a local Age Concern link, so you can contact a local office directly

Neurological Foundation of New Zealand
Ph: 09 309 7749
Fax: 09 377 0614
www.neurological.org.nz
admin@neurological.org.nz

Grey Power
National Office Ph: 09 277 7954
Fax: 09 277 7958
www.greypower.co.nz
fed-office@xtra.co.nz

Residential Care

Residential Information Services (Auckland and Northland)
Ph: 0800 725 463 or 09 375 4395
www.adhb.govt.nz/rcline

WINZ Residential Care Subsidy
Ph: 0800 997 727
www.workandincome.govt.nz
(more information on www.moh.govt.nz/assettesting

For people with dementia

Dementia Advocacy and Support Network
www.dasninternational.org

For information and support

Caring Caller and Lifelink medical alarm
National Office Ph: 04 472 3600
Fax: 04 498 2320
www.stjohn.org.nz
enquiries@stjohn.org.nz

Support for caregivers

Carers New Zealand
Ph: 09 406 0412
Fax: 09 406 1036
www.carers.net.nz
info@carers.net.nz

Gay and lesbian carers (UK):
Ph: 0044 207306 0606
www.alzheimers.org.uk/gay_carers
gaycarers@alzheimers.org.uk

Physical

Hip protectors
Ph/fax: 09 627 9596
www.impactwear.co.nz
info@impactwear.co.nz

Prevention

http://www.yourbrainmatters.org.au/

Treatment

The GM Resource and Referral Directory
www.gmd.net.nz
Counsellors, psychotherapists and other forms of therapy

New Zealand Society for Music Therapy
Ph: 04 234 7521
www.musictherapy.org.nz
To find a qualified music therapist

Medication

Janssen Cilag: (galantamine, risperidone) 0800 800 806
Pfizer: (donepezil) 0800 699 276 or 09 638 0000 or Apotex NZ Ltd 09 444 2073
Novartis: (rivastigmine) 09 828 3149
Pharmacia: 0800 276 520

Elder Abuse

Age Concern New Zealand
National Office Ph: 04 801 9338
Fax: 04 801 9336
www.ageconcern.org.nz
Elder abuse and neglect prevention service

Government Departments

Financial

WINZ Extra financial assistance: 0800 552 002
Community Service Card Info: 0800 999 999; or try website to print out an application form (www.workandincome.govt.nz)
Disability Allowance: 0800 559 009

Driving Assessment

For information on the closest assessment centre,
Enable New Zealand: 0800 171 981
And for fact sheets on medical conditions relating to driving: 0800 699 000 or www.ltsa.govt.nz

Health and Disability Commissioner

Freephone: 0800 112 233
Ph Auckland: 09 373 1060
Ph Wellington: 04 494 7900
www.hdc.org.nz
hdc@hdc.org.nz

Privacy Commissioner

Ph: 0800 803 909
Fax: 09 302 2305
www.privacy.org.nz

Ministry of Health

Ph: 04 496 2000
Fax: 04 496 2340
www.moh.govt.nz

Ministry of Justice

Ph: 04 918 8800
Fax: 04 918 8820
www.courts.govt.nz
reception@justice.govt.nz

Special Groups

The Stroke Foundation

Ph: 0800 STROKE (0800 78 76 53)

www.stroke.org.nz

strokenz@stroke.org.nz

Field officers, education, support groups, stroke club, research, information

Intellectually Handicapped Children's Society (IHC)

Ph: 04 471 6564

Fax: 04 472 0429

www.ihc.org.nz

Information on intellectual disability

Huntington's disease

www.hdlighthouse.org

Parkinson's New Zealand

Ph: 0800 4 PD INFO (0800 473 4636)

www.parkinsons.org.nz

Selected reading list

Bayley, John, *Iris: A Memoir of Iris Murdoch*, Duckworth Publications, London, 1998

Boden, Christine, *Who Will I Be When I Die?*, HarperCollins, Sydney, 1997

Davis, Robert, *My Journey into Alzheimer's Disease*, Tyndale House Publishers, Wheaton, Illinois, 1989

Forster, Margaret, *Have the Men Had Enough?*, Chatto & Windus, London, 1989

Reference books

Alzheimer's New Zealand Incorporated, *Dementia Economic Impact Report 2008*, Wellington, Access Economics for Alzheimer's New Zealand Incorporated, 2008. Retrieved from http://alzheimers.org.nz/assets/Uploads/AlzheimersReport2008.pdf in May 2012.

Garratt, Sally & Hamilton-Smith, Elery (eds.), *Rethinking Dementia: An Australian Approach*, Ausmed Publications, Melbourne, 1995

James, Oliver, *Contented Dementia: 24-hour Wraparound Care for Lifelong Wellbeing*, Ebury Press, London, 2010

Mace, Nancy L. & Rabins, Peter V., *The 36-Hour Day: A Family Guide to Caring for Persons with Alzheimer's Disease, Related Dementing Illnesses, and Memory Loss in Later Life*, rev. ed., Warner Books, New York, 2001

Ministry of Health, *Dementia in New Zealand: Improving Quality in Residential Care*, A report to the Disability Issues Directorate, January 2002

Ministry of Health, *The Health and Wellbeing of Older People and Kaumatua: the Public Health Issues*, Wellington, December 1997

Ministry of Health, *Mental Health and Addiction Services for Older People and Dementia Services: Guideline for district health boards on an integrated approach to mental health and addiction services for older people and dementia services for people of any age*, Wellington, Ministry of Health, 2011.

National Advisory Committee on Health and Disability, *Guidelines for the*

Support and Management of People with Dementia, Alzheimer's New Zealand (Ministry of Health), Wellington, reissued July 2003

Samuel, David, *Memory: How We Use it, Lose it, and Can Improve it*, New York University Press, New York, 1999

Sargeant, Delys & Unkenstein, Anne, *Remembering Well: How Memory Works and What To Do When It Doesn't*, Allen & Unwin, Sydney, 2nd ed., 2001

Stokes, Graham, *And Still the Music Plays*, 2nd ed., Hawker Publications, London, 2010

Stokes, Graham, *Challenging Behaviour in Dementia: A Person-centred Approach*, Speech Mark Publishing Ltd, Milton Keynes, 2000.

Taylor, Richard, *Alzheimer's from the Inside Out*, Health Professional Press Inc., Baltimore, 2007

Working Together We Can Respond to Dementia: Future directions for services, A report prepared by New Zealand Council of Christian Social Services, September 2009, http://www.nzccss.org.nz/uploads/publications/NZCCSSdementiareportFINAL29Sep09.pdf.

Children's information

Talking to children about your illness

www.alzheimers.org.uk/site/scripts/download_info.php?fileID=734.

Information about dementia for young people

www.fightdementia.org.au/understanding-dementia/section-6-young-people-and-dementia.aspx.

Other information

Brain donation

Many people suffering from Alzheimer's disease and their families would like to contribute to ongoing research into dementia. People in the Auckland area who wish to consider brain donation can contact Professor Richard Faull, Auckland Medical School, Park Rd, Grafton, and the Medical School will send out a *donor pack* to fill in. This gives details about the procedures to follow once the person with Alzheimer's disease dies. Only people from the Auckland area can contribute, and these people should have been through a specialist service to confirm the diagnosis of Alzheimer's disease (not other sorts of dementia). Because there are only limited facilities for this research, the offer of donation may not be accepted but is always appreciated.

Index